D1569274

The Electrophysiology of
Intellectual Functions

Duilio Giannitrapani

The Electrophysiology of Intellectual Functions

with a contribution by *W.T. Liberson*

32 figures and 55 tables, 1985

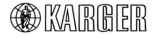

S. Karger · Basel · München · Paris · London · New York · Tokyo · Sydney

Duilio Giannitrapani, PhD

Veterans Administration Medical Center, Perry Point, Md., USA

formerly Director of Human Psychophysiology, Psychosomatic and Psychiatric Institute, Michael Reese Medical Center, Chicago, Ill., USA

National Library of Medicine, Cataloging in Publication
Giannitrapani, Duilio
The electrophysiology of intellectual functions/Duilio Giannitrapani; with a contribution by
W.T. Liberson. – Basel; New York: Karger, 1985.
Includes bibliographies and index.
1. Brain – physiology   2. Electroencephalography   3. Electrophysiology
I. Liberson, W.T., 1904–   II. Title
WL 300 G433e
ISBN 3–8055–3878–2

© Copyright 1985 by S. Karger AG, P.O. Box, CH–4009 Basel (Switzerland)
Printed in Switzerland by Thür AG Offsetdruck, Pratteln
ISBN 3–8055–3878–2

Contents

W.T. Liberson

IV Factor Analysis of the EEG

Foreword

It was with pleasure that I accepted the invitation to write a foreword for Dr. *Giannitrapani's* monograph on *The Electrophysiology of Intellectual Functions* and consider it a privilege for several reasons. One is related to the fact that Dr. *Giannitrapani,* an undergraduate student then, was first exposed to EEG at the Neuropsychiatric Institute in Hartford, Connecticut, where I was director of a laboratory of clinical neurophysiology. It was there that the term 'functional electroencephalography' was born. It was then that our laboratory was involved in the problems of intelligence and EEG, using, however, much less sophisticated analysis than that introduced to this field by Dr. *Giannitrapani.* Indeed, a second reason for enthusiastically endorsing his present effort is to acknowledge his personal contribution to the expansion of the frontiers of functional electroencephalography, taking advantage of the modern techniques of frequency and computerized factorial analyses of hidden aspects of brain waves simultaneously recorded from a number of scalp electrodes.

Dr. *Giannitrapani's* analysis of hidden information that is embedded in EEG tracings and which he so skilfully extracts clearly reveals the short-sightedness of those skeptics who claim that contributions of EEG are all but exhausted. In fact, these contributions have yet to be revealed to the majority of investigators by the type of new techniques of averaging, frequency and phase analysis and statistical studies, some of which are used by Dr. *Giannitrapani* in dealing with the crucial problems related to testing intelligence. He demonstrates that EEG is not merely a succession of sinusoidal-like wave forms but, in fact, contains a wealth of information unseen by the naked eye and which is to be extracted by the above-mentioned specific techniques. He conducted experiments at rest and during specific mental tasks and derived significant correlations with different aspects of human intellectual manifestations and performance.

A third and no less important reason for endorsing his monograph is that the material presented is bound to stimulate further thinking and research in the directions suggested by the author. Indeed, the value of any scientific work is not only in its immediate results but also in the hypotheses that it suggests and in the soundness of the investigative methodology that it uses. I, for my part, took advantage of the data that I extracted from Dr. *Giannitrapani's* experimental work to complement my old thesis of the role played by the activating function of the brain stem on intellectual performance (see chapter 13).

It seems certain that neurophysiologists, psychologists and physicians will all find it of great interest. All in all, I trust that Dr. *Giannitrapani's* monograph will be a milestone in the modern development of 'functional electroencephalography'.

W.T. Liberson, MD, PhD
Past President, American Electroencephalographic Society

Foreword

Some years ago as Chairman of the Department of Psychiatry at Michael Reese Hospital in Chicago, I invited Dr. *Giannitrapani* to be Director of Human Psychophysiology. Slowly and systematically he developed a methodology founded on EEG spectral analysis which enabled him to isolate a specific type of schizophrenia difficult for the clinician to understand.

But behind this first approach to a relationship between neurophysiology and clinical disease was a forerunner of a new type of testing for mental abilities and disease by objective physiological measures, rather than verbal responses, developing a new approach to clinical diagnosis. The link between EEG and mental properties is thus established which redefines intellectual functions on the basis of electrophysiological parameters rather than on speculation based on nonobjective psychological tests. Mentation, healthy and sick, is related closely to patterns of neural activity demonstrated clearly by a wide variety of experiments not easily understood by the clinician.

Until recently we have isolated the psychological test data as a reductionistic isolated function. Physiological data derived from human EEG studies has likewise been reductionistic. Now *Giannitrapani* has brought the two together as a unitary system of component parts regulated and controlled to maintain equilibrium and integration. Substance essential to these processes casts a new perspective on living processes.

Giannitrapani's work is highly sophisticated, a necessity which permitted him to link physiology and mental phenomena into parts of a total system. The technique may be unfamiliar to the clinician, but the results are the important factor and give meaning to what in nature is a process.

Roy R. Grinker, Sr., MD

Founder and Director Emeritus, Psychosomatic and Psychiatric Institute, Michael Reese Medical Center, Chicago, Ill.

Preface

If there was a beginning it was in 1944 when at the age of 17 I began arguing with myself whether animals had intelligence. After spending the summer in the library, I wrote a treatise with the conclusion that the answer depended on one's definition of intelligence. The search for this definition and the search for the facts upon which to base it constitute the warp of my quest.

At about that time there was another beginning. In 1945, *Roy R. Grinker, Sr.* accomplished his aim of founding a research institute in conjunction with a psychiatric institute. At the inauguration ceremonies of the Psychosomatic and Psychiatric Institute for Research and Training of Michael Reese Hospital, *Percival Bailey* spoke about higher cortical functions and their genesis. He invoked the then in vogue scanning mechanism construct.

In 1947, the woof of my quest took a physiological bent when I met Dr. *W.T. Liberson* in his EEG laboratory full of tube-type amplifiers of that vintage, became fascinated with the EEG technique and asked him about intelligence. His brusque rebuff, perhaps due to his frustrations in his search for EEG correlates of higher cortical functions, did not reveal the fact that indeed he was a pioneer in this quest.

19 years later, *Bailey's* hopes, the woof of my quest and *Grinker's* vision converged when Dr. *Grinker* offered me the opportunity to establish the human psychophysiology laboratory at P & PI. This book represents some of the work conducted there between 1966 and 1971 with the benefit of subsequent thinking and analyses performed with partial support of the Veterans Administration at Perry Point.

Duilio Giannitrapani, PhD
Perry Point, Md.

Acknowledgements

I am indebted, first to my wife, *Corinne,* for firmly believing – even when I didn't – that the only difference between my dreams and reality was just a matter of time.

I am indebted to *Roy R. Grinker, Sr.* who bought the dream; to *Donald O. Walter* who made an easy path of spectral analysis for the dream; to *Bernard Saltzberg* for teaching math to the dream; to Pivan Engineering, *Will Rast* and *Bud Schulhafer* for translating my dream into a hardware-feasible concept; to *Franklin Offner* who reintroduced and insisted on a 17th monitoring channel to guarantee that the dream was based on facts; to *Peter Roccaforte* for getting the hardware to work without losing sight of the dream and for being a valuable collaborator; to *Richard Snekhaus, Neal Kuhn* and *Bill Clusin* for programming the dream and skilfully guiding the data through various computers; to *Bill Clusin* also for help in designing the psychological variables for the dream and, with *Ralph Cady,* for administering all the psychological testing to the children of the dream; to *Enoch Calloway* for furnishing a full carton of IBM cards of A/D conversions for checking out the newly developed computer programs; to *Neil Palmer* for his armchair wisdom; to *Ed Barnes* who taught me the first law of creativity: to find the simplest path; to *Constance Bailey* who, with a smile, ran all the EEGs for the dream; to *Garnett Pace* and *Sheryl Braggio* for sorting through the data; to my daughter *Laura* for the art work to make it a pleasing dream; to *James Gargiulo,* my son *Robert, Luciano L'Abate, Cathryn Walters Liberson, W.T. Liberson* and *Sonoko Ohwaki* for valuable comments about the manuscript; to my wife for editing and typing the manuscript; to my daughter *Diana* for proofreading and indexing; and to *Paul Stickler* for being a friend throughout.

At the Veterans Administration Medical Center in Perry Point, Maryland, I am indebted to *Edward Sieracki* and *Lee Crump* for their support of my research effort; to *James Klett, Joe Collins* and *Rod Gillis* for the generous help of the VA Cooperative Studies Center in accomplishing the factor analysis of the EEG; to *James Gargiulo* for data analysis; to *Luther Gilliam* and *Donna Asher* for the layout and photography of the artwork; and to *Elizabeth McMillan,* librarian, for her invaluable assistance.

Finally to the staff of Karger for their superb handling of the author and of the manuscript.

This research was supported in part by USPHS Grant No. MH5519 and by the Veterans Administration.

Grateful acknowledgment for copyright permission is made to the following (appropriate credits are made in the text where applicable): Fischer (Stuttgart); The Psychological Corporation (New York); Plenum (New York); *Behavioral Science* (Houston, Tex.).

To *Heinz Werner*

I Electrophysiology of Mental Abilities

'... the approach of making up subjective armchair definitions of intelligence is foredoomed, logically and methodologically.'
R.B. Cattell

1 Introduction

'Has the brain explained the mind? If it has, does the brain do so by the simple performance of its neuronal mechanisms, or by the supplying of energy to the mind? Or both? Does it supply the mind with energy and at the same time provide it with basic neuronal mechanisms that are related to consciousness?'
Wilder Penfield

The study of mental abilities is limited to our current understanding of mental functions. This understanding governs current theories which in turn determine what is accepted as fact. The existence of relationships between electrocortical brain activity and scores of currently used mental ability measures is studied for the purpose of furthering the understanding of mental abilities and the mechanisms governing their mediation in the brain. The relationships that were found to exist between mental abilities and brain activity studied via frequency analysis of the electroencephalogram (EEG) are explored in this book.

There are two landmarks in the progress of scientific thought in the field of mental abilities. The first is *Spearman's* [1927] application of Pearson's correlation technique which marked the beginning of the replacement of armchair speculation with mathematical arguments. Prior to the advent of the correlation method, the degree of independence of different mental faculties or abilities was strictly a matter of conjecture. *Spearman* [1904] had first introduced Pearson's product-moment correlation method into psychology when he postulated (and later was able to demonstrate) the existence of a general intelligence component (a factor common to all faculties), as well as more specific components, factors which he found to be specific to the different functions involved. The second landmark is the development by *Thurstone* [1935, 1938] of the factor analytic method which consists of an in-depth analysis of intercorrelation matrices. He applied this method to the field of evaluating mental abilities.

These two techniques removed the study of mental abilities from the field of pure conjecture and placed it in a realm founded on actual computations, giving the word 'factor' a statistical mathematical meaning. Placing the discussion of mental abilities on the mathematical level, however, did not eliminate the problems. It succeeded instead in replacing arguments having the intrinsic logic of face validity with arguments in hyperspace in which multiple factors could be conceived.

With spectral analysis of the EEG, the study of mental abilities was retrieved from hyperspace and returned to a realm closer to a meaningful relationship with the organism, i.e. by determining the relationship of these mathematically derived constructs to the electrophysiological activity of the brain.

The measurement of mental abilities has been restricted almost exclusively to behavioral correlates obtained by performance on selected intellectual tasks. Since intelligence is a process that cannot be measured directly, it is inferred at the present time from scores obtained through performance on verbal/behavioral tests. This process is still considered broadly unidimensional. Through standardization of the responses in a population sample, a given score is statistically related to a degree of difficulty, and these scores, weighted and normalized, are transformed into scores which are used as indicators of the intellectual capacity of a given subject.

The major drawback of this method is the inferential step between the mental functions the individual is capable of performing (process) and the scores (outcome). The present investigation is an attempt to remove that inferential step in the measurement of mental abilities, i.e. to test the validity of a process measure (EEG scores) to eliminate the intervening behavioral component altogether. These tests are used primarily to attempt an understanding of the electrophysiological variables that may either preside over or constitute the sine qua non of intellectual functions and secondarily to evaluate the validity of behavioral intelligence tests.

The study of a number of electrophysiological variables in each of a number of cortical brain areas provides the dimensionality required for detecting the diverse functional roles of cortical structures as well as those of electrophysiological parameters. With this approach, intelligence loses its unidimensionality which is replaced by functions having electrophysiological validity. The possibility of studying these new functions, some of which may have been recognized already by psychology, and others, for which there is no current understanding, denotes a major progress in the measurement of mental abilities.

During the past 40 years the anticipation of the establishment of a link between electroencephalography and mental properties has been the underlying rationale for the study of electrocortical activity. The earliest investigators knew that mental activity had profound effects on scalp electricity. Subsequent investigators had relatively little success in their attempts to understand the nature of cortical potentials in the study of cortical-mentation relationships. Very little systematic work has occurred in determining which aspects of intellectual behavior are concurrent with physiological activity as measured by the EEG.

The present investigation was founded on the assumption that the human cortex is organized in some measurable fashion for the performance of abstract intellectual tasks. The theory that EEG is attributable to gross synchronization of synaptic potentials and to circulation of impulses in closed self-reexciting chains, articulated by *Eccles* [1951], has not been replaced by a more viable alternative [for current thinking on the subject, cf. *Nunez*, 1981]. The mentation-EEG correlates observed in the present study are postulated to be determined by paths of different duration for circulating impulses consequent to changing background levels of neuronal activity. They are interpreted as surface traits and should furnish the needed motivation for initiating additional neurophysiologically oriented studies. Furthermore, the existence of these correlates opens a new area of investigation, i.e. the redefining of intellectual functions on the basis of electrophysiological parameters rather than on the basis of armchair speculation or pragmatic statistics as is currently done.

This book succeeds in its task to a measurable degree. It demonstrates the existence of certain EEG components which do not alter their relationship with mental abilities while the subject is engaging in a broad variety of activities. These EEG components, therefore, are closer to the process than to behavior as in the case of traditional mental ability tests.

A further elaboration of the data through a series of factor analyses permits moving from the level of surface trait to source trait [*Cattell,* 1971] by mapping the scalp distribution of EEG frequency components which load a single factor, i.e. which contribute to a single electrophysiologically derived function.

Since the cortex is a multifunction structure, in the course of electrocortical mapping of functions, other variables which may interact with mental activity need to be studied. Some such variables are brain dominance, perceptual processing, age of the subject and, as observed late in the study, the sex of the subject. Attention, therefore, needs to be given to these variables.

The findings of this study represent a major attempt to date to reach an understanding of mental abilities as they are organized in the brain. These data help reorganize the concept of mental abilities on an electrophysiological basis, thereby removing one more veil that prevents us from seeing the mind and brain as one.

The organization of the book is as follows:

Part I introduces the problem, history and method used including details of technical and theoretical considerations of the spectral analysis technique for prospective investigators. It also includes a reliability study which was performed to determine the degree of confidence that could be placed in this data.

Part II introduces the first analyses of both autospectral and cross-spectral data, showing the sensitivity and dimensionality of this methodology for this type of investigation. The issues of the lateralization of the findings and brain dominance are discussed here.

Part III presents the bulk of the data with an analysis of the various matrices of correlations obtained between EEG and mental abilities as well as between EEG and intellectual factor scores. Interpretation and points of comparison with clinical data, tapping primarily the current neuropsychological understanding of the field, are made whenever applicable.

Chapter 13 presents Dr. *Liberson's* interpretation of the data. In order to analyze it along the unidimension, active-passive intelligence, he averaged brain areas, frequency bands and WISC subtests. My bias is to refrain from conceptualizing intelligence as a unidimensional function and also to refrain from conceptualizing EEG as consisting of broad frequency bands or of brain hemispheres as functioning as a unit. Dr. *Liberson's* approach, beyond the intrinsic value of his findings, is of great consequence as it constitutes another example of how hypotheses of the structure of intelligence can be tested against physiological criteria.

Part IV introduces the factor analyses performed on the EEG data in order to gain a better understanding of the role the different frequencies and brain areas have in the performance of higher cortical functions.

Part V presents a neurophysiological interpretation of the data within a scanning theory framework and summarizes the findings.

References

Cattell, R.B.: Abilities: their structure, growth and action (Houghton Mifflin, Boston 1971).

Eccles, J.C.: Interpretation of action potentials evoked in the cerebral cortex. Electroenceph. clin. Neurophysiol. *3:* 449–464 (1951).

Nunez, P.L.: Electric fields of the brain, the neurophysics of EEG (Oxford University Press, New York 1981).

Spearman, C.: General intelligence objectively determined and measured. Am. J. Psychol. *15:* 201–293 (1904).

Spearman, C.: The abilities of man, pp. 448 (Macmillan, London 1927).

Thurstone, L.L.. The factorial isolation of primary abilities. Psychometrika *1:* No. 3 (1935).

Thurstone, L.L.: Primary mental abilities. Psychometric Monogr., No. 1, pp. v–121 (University of Chicago Press, Chicago 1938).

2 History of EEG-Mental Ability Studies

'Difficult problems like the nature of thinking and memory are approached
from two directions, through neurophysiological methods – studying the
physics, chemistry, and biology of the nerve systems – and through
psychological methods – studying the observed phenomena in the brain.
This research can be thought of as boring a tunnel from two sides: the two
approaches have not yet met but hopefully some day they will.'
B. Weisskopf

Mental activity is so different from any other body function that even
today it is given an implied extracorporeal status. It was only recently that
some of the higher functions were transposed from the heart to the brain.
Hippocrates observed contralateral motor-function deficits with head injuries but did not gain an understanding of the function of the central nervous
system nor of contralaterality and much less of the nature of mentation.
During the succeeding 2,000 years the world of ideas has preceded the
world of demonstrations, and today one generally accepts that the mind is
in the brain even though, as *Eccles* [1951] pointed out, we do not have any
scientific evidence for such a statement. The research for the understanding
of brain functions has recapitulated the phylogenetic progression from
motor to speech, leaving at present large unexplored cortical areas euphe-
mistically identified as silent or association areas.

The performance of abstract intellectual tasks requires a mental organization which should have direct neural correlates [the theoretical and
philosophical state of the art is best exemplified by *Eccles,* 1976]. This has
been an implicit assumption in neuorological cognitive studies which have
attempted to detect principles of 'information processing'.

The neurophysiological studies dealing with synaptic 'learning', inhib-
itory and excitatory postsynaptic potentials and gross synchronization of
synaptic potentials are exciting per se and have provided very much needed

information, but they are not expected to furnish, in the very near future, an understanding of complex brain functions. For the latter, a noninvasive method such as multiple-channel EEG is needed for investigation of more global processes.

Alpha Activity Studies

The earliest investigators in EEG, including *Berger* in 1938 [*Gloor,* 1969], hypothesized that cognitive functions could be detected through electrocortical potentials. The idea that electrophysiological output is a correlate of mental ability is founded in the notion that mentation is consequent to patterns of neural activity with their necessary chemical and electrophysiological correlates. *Berger* in 1932 began by observing a reduction in amplitude and frequency of alpha rhythm among the severely retarded, and later in 1938 [*Gloor,* 1969] he observed among mature adult mentally defectives more regular alpha rhythm than in younger normal adults. He described how the alpha rhythm in mentally defective subjects is more representative of a 'resting condition' than the rhythm of a normal subject. He suggested, therefore, that alpha activity, rather than describing a resting state, would be better identified as portraying a brain in a 'passive' state as contrasted with the 'active' brain in which alpha disappears and beta or faster activity increases.

Even though this analysis is incomplete in light of present knowledge, the inference is that in the resting state of a normal subject some cerebral activity is always present, activity which modulates the alpha rhythm with a superimposition of faster activity.

Subsequent studies of EEG and intelligence grew out of the investigation of mentally deficient subjects. They have been of limited value because a given EEG abnormality can occur with a multitude of etiological factors.

In a group of Down's syndrome subjects *Kreezer* [1939] found a correlation (rho = 0.35) between mental age and the alpha index (percent time alpha). He found no such correlation in a group of retarded non-Down's syndrome subjects, but he did find in the latter a significant correlation (0.32) between mental age and alpha frequency. After several experiments, *Kreezer and Smith* [1950] concluded that there was a weak but appreciable positive correlation betwen alpha frequency and mental age in a group of adult nondifferentiated familial type mentally retarded.

Extending the research to a normal sample of 9-year-olds, *Knott* et al. [1942] found a correlation of 0.50 between occipital alpha frequency and intelligence quotient (IQ). Unfortunately, the same comparison was not significant for a group of 12-year-olds. The authors attributed this to an inadequate handling of statistics. Although the correlation for 12-year-olds fails to reach the significance level of the first correlation, it should be noted that the difference between the two is also not significant ($p > 0.2$ by the Z' test). These discoveries tended to be ephemeral. In similar studies, *Lindsley* [1938], *Henry* [1944] and *Shagass* [1946] found no significant correlation with either alpha frequency or alpha index.

Mundy-Castle [1958], the first investigator to study EEG and intellectual variables utilizing factor analysis, demonstrated in a group of normal adults a relationship between alpha frequency and Wechsler-Bellevue Vocabulary ($r = 0.406$), Object Assembly ($r = 0.413$), Verbal IQ ($r = 0.417$), Performance IQ ($r = 0.403$) and Full-Scale IQ ($r = 0.507$). He also found relationships between alpha index (amplitude) and Wechsler-Bellevue Arithmetic ($r = 0.475$), Picture Completion ($r = 0.434$) and Picture Arrangement ($r = 0.413$). These data point to the independence of alpha frequency and alpha index reaffirmed by the factor structure found by *Mundy-Castle* [1958]. Alpha frequency shows a positive loading (0.418) and alpha index a negative loading (−0.332) on factor A, a factor otherwise loaded on performance subtests (a type III factor in the present study, cf. table 12/IV). Alpha frequency [*Mundy-Castle*, 1958] also shows a positive loading (0.502) on factor D, a numerical factor which loads on Arithmetic and Digit Span, while alpha index has its only strong positive loading (0.665) on factor B, another numerical factor which loads in addition on Block Design (both having a type I factor pattern in our study, cf. table 12/II and chapter 12 for a fuller discussion of Wechsler Intelligence Scale for Children, WISC, factor analysis studies).

Netchine and Lairy [1960, 1962] explained the elusive character of the correlations between EEG activity and mental ability scores by pointing out that high alpha frequencies can also occur among young subjects of low intelligence. As a result, the frequencies of the low intelligence group have a greater range (6–14 Hz) than the middle or higher IQ groups. This might be due to a greater heterogeneity in the degree of brain dysfunction in the population of low intelligence. *Netchine and Lairy* [1960, 1962] also developed an 'S' index dealing with the amplitudes of alpha activity in the occipital, parietal and rolandic areas. Some relatively complex relationships between these different measures and intelligence were demonstrated.

In the present investigation, dominant alpha frequency was studied by obtaining for each subject an average (for the 8 conditions) of the magnitude of the power spectral values of the 2 occipital derivations in the 4 frequency bands (2 Hz wide) from 6 to 14 Hz. The frequency band with the highest average power was assumed to represent the dominant frequency for that subject. If 2 adjacent frequency bands were approximately of the same value, a frequency value in between the 2 frequency bands was used to represent the dominant alpha frequency for that subject. In the computation of the rhos, because of the many ties, a formula with correction for ties was used.

To determine whether a correlation between alpha frequency and age was evident in this age group (a span of 3 years), a correlation was performed between the two variables. The rho = +0.04 indicates no relationship between alpha frequency and age in this group of 11- to 13-year-olds. This finding is in accord with the observations of *Lindsley* [1938, 1939] and *Smith* [1938, 1941] who found no appreciable change in alpha frequency in the age range of the present study.

The correlation between the same dominant alpha frequency scores and WISC Full-Scale IQ was also calculated. A rho = +0.44 was obtained, indicating a positive and significant relationship between dominant alpha frequency and IQ as observed by earlier investigators.

To study the correlation between dominant alpha index and IQ in the present investigation, the power spectral density values of the 9- and 11-Hz bands in the occipital areas were added to form a single score which included all the activity from 8 to 12 Hz. These scores, separate for left and right occipital, were correlated against the 3 main WISC IQ scores. All of the correlations obtained were positive, but the 0.05 level of significance was reached only with Performance IQ in the left occipital area (rho = +0.24).

Previous work with an adult sample by the present investigator [*Giannitrapani,* 1969] also demonstrated higher correlations with Performance IQ. In conclusion, there seems to be a relationship between both alpha variables and IQ but alpha frequency and alpha index account for a different portion of the variance as demonstrated by the inverse realtionship in the growth curve of the 2 phenomena as shown by *Lindsley* [1939] and more directly demonstrated by the independence of the factor loadings of the 2 parameters in *Mundy-Castle's* [1958] factor analysis. The identification of the respective components remains to be determined and may not be possible until a better understanding of the nature of alpha activity is reached.

Disease Entity Studies

Liberson made several attempts to find EEG parameters relating to intelligence. In addition to his PhD thesis [1950], he studied [1951] the relationships between several EEG variables and intellectual deterioration among mentally ill patients. He found characteristic homologous asymmetries in the distribution of alpha activity and quickly came to the conclusion that an EEG conceptual index would have to take into account the age variable. *Liberson* [1967] published a comprehensive review of EEG abnormalities in mentally defective subjects. Considering in detail such tendencies as the excessive theta (2–7 Hz) rhythms, he concluded that normal intellect and normal EEG are both manifestations of the same physiological state. Unfortunately, his lines of investigation have not been pursued with normal subjects, and it is difficult to extract normal parameters from research with samples of defectives. A comprehensive attempt to review EEG frequency findings relating to conceptualization and pathology was made by *Walters* [1964].

While studying a specific syndrome, *Gastaut* et al. [1968] reasserted the occurrence of serious mental retardation in juvenile epileptic encephalopathy associated with diffuse slow spike wave activity (Lennox syndrome). Major etiological factors listed constitute quite a broad spectrum and are, in order of importance, perinatal trauma, postnatal acute encephalopathy and heredity. One other such investigation was made by *Hagberg and Sjögren* [1968] on infantile hydrocephalus. They indicated that the presence of a given disease process is not a sufficient condition for mental impairment.

In another group of studies, investigators selected a specific kind of mentally impaired subjects and sought clinical correlates. In one study *Seppalainen and Kivalo* [1967] studied a group of Down's syndrome subjects and established that severe EEG abnormality was common but varied. They observed diffuse cortical disturbance, paroxysmal activity and epilepsy, listed in order of importance.

Attempts to gain information about EEG correlates of mental ability from traditional clinical EEG studies, disease entity studies and mental retardation studies share the shortcoming of relying on a common factor (a given EEG abnormality, a given disease entity, or a given type of intellectual deficit) which is never found to occur in conjunction with a single set of determinants.

To deal with the question of abnormality in low intelligence subjects,

Gibbs et al. [1960] surveyed a large population having low IQ. They found an increasing percentage of EEG abnormalities as the IQ diminished.

Other studies using EEG indices having developmental significance also dealt with only one EEG variable. *Jenkins* [1962], for instance, found a relationship between the presence of EEG slow activity and impaired performance on sensory motor tests, but historically the major thrust was directed at exploring alpha activity.

A single EEG measure such as alpha amplitude, alpha frequency or presence of slow activity cannot be expected to fully represent a low IQ condition which varies on so many dimensions, i.e. age, type of mental defect, etiology, age of onset, and last but not least, association with other abnormalities.

In summary, the bulk of the findings attempting to deal with the relationships between EEG and mental abilities were extrapolations of traditional EEG clinical parameters with their intrinsic medical pathological model, the notion being that EEG abnormalities were equated with brain disease, ergo low IQ. While it is unquestioned that brain disease affects perforce mental functioning, an understanding of the electrophysiology of mental activity is not necessarily obtained by studying the anomalous case.

This new quest for mental activity in the healthy brain does not rely on traditional EEG findings. In the absence of reliable precursors, this study was committed to a broad-spectrum search unfettered by clinical preconceptions. It was decided that if in the course of the investigation traditional clincical parameters were found to relate to the variables in question, they would be discussed in order to further clinical EEG knowledge.

Evoked Potential Studies

The availability of instrumentation for electronic averaging has encouraged recent interest in studying the effects of perceptual stimulation on EEG patterns. The shape of the averaged potential can be examined either as to the time lags of its different components or by Fourier analysis of the evoked wave form.

There are some limitations inherent in the evoked potential technique. It is restricted to the study of average EEG activity elicited by repetitive stimulation, activity which is known to change with each repetition. It studies a brief electrical potential (consequent to stimulation) which shows a great similarity in all brain areas and is therefore not the most sensitive to study the functioning of different brain areas.

The limitations of the evoked potential method are such that their latency scores may be useful in the context of a reaction time paradigm and its contribution to intellectual functioning but not to further the understanding of the complex attributes of intelligence.

While it is outside the scope of this publication to critically review the literature dealing with evoked potentials and their relationships with intellectual functions, inconsistent evoked potential findings may be due to several factors among which are: (1) use of only 1 or 2 leads, not necessarily comparable between studies; (2) difficulty in identifying the initial evoked potential component; (3) the effect of differences in the state of attention or arousal [*Shucard and Horn,* 1972]; and (4) in the case of latency measures, the variability introduced by the portion of the phase of the alpha cycle in which triggering occurred [*Dustman and Beck,* 1965].

A development of the evoked potential studies in this field consists of Fourier analysis of the evoked potential. This procedure was suggested by *Walter* [*Adey,* 1969] as an attempt to obtain spectral EEG measurements of short duration with an increased reliability over steady-state EEG. In this group of studies, *Weinberg* [1969] found a correlation between verbal IQ and the presence of 12–14 Hz activity in 500 ms of visual evoked potential data. *Osaka and Osaka* [1980], also with spectral analysis of evoked potentials, found a peak at 12 Hz in normal subjects as compared with mentally retarded subjects. The group of frequencies included in what the authors referred to as 12-Hz activity is not identified in their publication. It could include, therefore, the frequencies responsible for *Weinberg's* [1969] finding as well as the frequencies responsible for the 13-Hz findings of the present study obtained from steady-state EEG.

In light of the findings of the present study which demonstrated that an EEG steady-state 13-Hz component (12–14 Hz) is strongly related to verbal IQ [first reported at the Central Association of Electroencephalographers Meeting in Chicago, October 1970], evoked potential findings will be discussed further in chapter 18.

Developmental Theory

Another reason for studying intellectual functions via the EEG is given by the observation concerning the increase of the frequency of dominant activity with age [*Lindsley,* 1938]. Attempts to relate this developmental feature with intelligence met with limited success. For a brief history of studies on the relationship between alpha amplitude, alpha frequency and intelligence see *Giannitrapani* [1969]. Severe limitations were present in the hand scoring of the EEG records of these investigations.

Developmental theory [*Werner,* 1940] postulates an increase of differentiation and hierarchic integration both phylogenetically and ontogenetically. If this principle were to be invoked, it could be hypothesized that these processes would be reflected not only in intellectual performance but in the EEG scores as well. Lack of differentiation of functions among brain areas could be manifested in a greater homogeneity of activity obtained from different electrode placements in low IQ subjects.

It is for this reason that the present study, aimed at exploring the intellectual correlates of EEG activity in a broad spectrum of frequencies from 0 to 34 Hz, was subdivided into narrow bands. In effect, findings were sought by studying: (1) dominant alpha amplitude (alpha index); (2) amplitude of other frequency components perhaps occurring from a 'desynchronizing' process; (3) dominant alpha frequency; (4) incidence of EEG activity in a broad-frequency spectrum, and (5) relationships of the activity between brain areas.

The autospectra, which are proportional to the square of the amplitude, are used to deal with the first 4 questions, while the cross-spectra are used to measure the relationship of the activity between brain areas. Two additional sets of measures, phase angle and coherence, were obtained but are not discussed in this book. With the analysis of phase angle scores one can infer transmission lags between points in the cortex or between a common subcortical source and 2 points in the cortex.

Cross-spectra and coherence, instead, are different indicators of similarity of the activity of the 2 areas involved. As such they may reflect, in different ways along with autospectra, the degree of differentiation between brain areas. While phase angle and coherence were shown to be useful parameters in the discrimination of behavioral states, correlations with intellectual scores have not yet been performed.

Spectral Analysis and the Present Study

A first attempt to quantifiy a broad spectrum of EEG frequencies was made by *Giannitrapani and Stoddard* [1960] and *Giannitrapani* [1969] with a visual count of EEG frequencies in 20 subjects. It was not a frequency analysis as such, but a higher count indicated a relatively greater amount of fast activity. Results indicated that a $\frac{thinking}{resting}$ ratio was greater in the frontal and occipital lobes in all but 6 of 18 subjects, 3 of whom had an IQ of less than 100. Another finding was that all subjects with less than 100 IQ showed a greater $\frac{thinking}{resting}$ ratio in the parietal than in the occipital areas. Also, subjects who showed $\frac{thinking}{resting}$ ratios occipital > parietal > frontal had performance IQ > verbal IQ.

These findings indicated that frequency analysis was a fruitful research area for the study of the organization of electrophysiological activity relating to higher brain functions, but serious problems of instrumentation and methodology were present. The available electronic frequency analyzers with resonating filters were unreliable, and it could not be hypothesized a priori whether higher or lower EEG amplitude was a correlate of mental activity. It was known that a decrease in alpha activity and an increase in beta activity occurred with mentation. Since muscle electrical potential is known to cluster in the high beta band as well as in higher frequencies, a portion of the increase in beta in certain brain areas often had been attributed to muscle artifacts consequent to an assumed increase in muscle tone during mentation.

Investigations stemming from those of *Walter* [1943] depended upon electronic resonating filters that have unstable tuning characteristics. The nature of the filters was such that they responded best to repetitive waves. The most characteristic feature of the EEG, however, is that its frequency components are constantly changing so that the resonating filters were least sensitive to the largest portion of the ongoing activity.

The development of period analytic techniques for the analysis of EEG data dispelled some of the difficulties encountered by electronic spectral analysis. As a form of frequency analysis, the instrument used in period analysis, however, received a limited utilization. Introduced by *Saltzberg and Burch* [1957] and *Burch* [1959, 1964], interest shifted away from this technique with the advent of computerized spectral analysis even though it has been shown to be as effective as other more complex techniques [*Saltzberg and Burch*, 1971].

The possibility of reliably measuring the frequency components of the resulting complex wave forms was not present until digitizing, computer processing and a new algorithm for fast Fourier analysis became available.

High-speed electronic computers capable of handling a vastly greater amount of information have revolutionized the field of EEG inquiry

[*Brazier,* 1965] as they have other areas of endeavor. The availability and popularization of analogue-to-digital conversion systems permitted the Fourier analysis of EEG data by digital computer. This analysis, once a formidably long undertaking, was brought within practical use by the application of the *Cooley and Tukey* [1965] algorithm, considerably shortening the computations. Despite the possible advances in electroencephalography that could accrue from the use of computers, there has been a decided lag between available technology and its widespread use.

Systematic efforts have been made by this investigator who, during the past 20 years of research, has been engaged in the exploitation of the computer's capacities for the purposes of electroencephalography. There was a progression from the use of manual analysis in 1958 [*Giannitrapani,* 1966, 1969] to an unsuccessful attempt at electronic spectral analysis in 1959. After several years work with the electronic phase analyzers developed by Darrow [*Giannitrapani* et al., 1966], this investigator developed a system in which EEG signals are digitized at the time of data acquisition and simultaneously recorded on computer tape for the computation of autospectra at a later date [*Giannitrapani* et al., 1971].

An additional dimension of the EEG which became available with the advent of frequency analysis with the computer is the measurement of the relationship of the activity between different brain areas such as phase angle between brain areas and coherence. The usefulness of these scores in a broad spectrum of studies of brain functions has been amply demonstrated [*Walter* et al., 1966; *Giannitrapani,* 1975, 1979a, b].

Spectral analysis is not without pitfalls, and care must be taken in interpreting the high amplitude at the low frequency end of EEG spectral displays. The characteristic downward slope of spectral displays, not necessarily intrinsic to EEG signals, might be due to a number of reasons founded in the mathematics of Fourier analysis. *Giannitrapani* et al. [1983] demonstrated both empirically and mathematically that the presence of EEG frequencies of short duration and, in particular, of EEG activity of the duration of less than 1 Hz (fractional wave form) is not identified by the Fourier algorithms. It appears as an increase in power at the low end of the frequency spectrum.

The EEG signals have a characteristic nonstationarity, but to what extent fractional wave forms are responsible for this increase in power at the low end of the spectrum remains to be studied. The downward slope of an EEG spectral display may come to be regarded not as an artifact but as a meaningful parameter if individual differences in the production of EEG fractional wave forms would be found to be related to specific differences in brain mechanisms. There is some objection to adopting the term fractional wave form because it is not in the nature of biological phenomena for component frequencies to suddenly appear and disappear. This is not a real issue because the same problem exists for changes in amplitude of the signal of a given frequency, the problem becoming significant with more rapid changes in amplitude of the signal.

Another problem that arises when hypothesizing cross-spectral correlates of mentation is whether a high degree of synchrony or a high degree of asynchrony is a correlate of high intellectual function. It is being postulated that both conditions may occur in different brain areas and/or in different frequency bands and that it might be possible to differentiate among the components of a given function on this basis. The study of phase and coherence, however, is outside the scope of the present publication.

A physiological exploration into the area of mentation would have to be broadly based and use statistics of the two-tailed test type in order to detect the crucial parameters. It would be hoped that the data would have a certain amount of face validity, i.e. demonstrate specific relationships with the brain structures known to be involved in the performance of the functions subsumed by the criterion variable. Other findings involving structures with unknown functions could then be used to develop hypotheses and make further investigations.

At the inception of the present investigation, two methods were contemplated. In the first and more obvious one the EEG spectra would be obtained while the subject was performing the task under consideration. Any observed changes would be due to the task. The problem with this method is that the observed changes may be unrelated to the cognitive components of the task under investigation. An alternate method, which at first sight seems more inferential but which yields clearer results, is to obtain the spectra under conditions unrelated to the cognitive variable and correlate the EEG spectral values with the behavioral scores obtained for the cognitive task. This second method, which proved to be fruitful, assumes the presence at all times of EEG frequency components which correlate with conceptual activity. To appear, they do not need the triggering which occurs when the brain engages in conceptual activity.

One must also differentiate between mentation and the capacity for mentation. Certain EEG values which may be a correlate of mentation may be orthogonal or inversely related to a measure of the capacity or ability for engaging in mental activity.

The purpose of the present investigation is 3-fold: (1) to find electrophysiological components of intellectual functions; (2) with a multiple electrode technique, to determine which brain areas are involved in specific cognitive functions, and (3) to categorize cognitive functions in terms of their neurophysiological correlates in order to restructure our thinking about intellectual functions along neurophysiological dimensions.

To conclude, the present investigation differs significantly from early research by (1) utilizing EEG spectral analysis, (2) investigating the differential role of 16 brain areas, and (3) utilizing EEG measures which are unrelated to the intellectual tasks.

References

Adey, W.R.: Spectral analysis of EEG data from animals and man during alerting, orienting and discriminative responses; in Evans, Mulholland, Attention in neurophysiology, pp. 194–229 (Butterworth, London 1969).

Brazier, M.A.B.: The application of computers to electroencephalography; in Stacy, Waxman, Computers in biomedical research, vol. 1, pp. 295–315 (Academic Press, New York 1965).

Burch, N.R.: Automatic analysis of the electroencephalogram. A review and a classification of systems. Electroenceph. clin. Neurophysiol. *11:* 827–834 (1959).

Burch, N.R.: Period analysis of the EEG on a general-purpose digital computer. Ann. N.Y. Acad. Sci. *115:* 827–843 (1964).

Cooley, J.W.; Tukey, J.W.: An algorithm for the machine calculation of complex Fourier series. Math. Comp. *19:* 297–301 (1965).

Dustman, R.E.; Beck, E.C.: Phase of alpha brain waves, reaction time and visually evoked potentials. Electroenceph. clin. Neurophysiol. *18:* 433–440 (1965).

Eccles, J.C.: Interpretation of action potentials evoked in the cerebral cortex. Electroenceph. clin. Neurophysiol. *3:* 449–464 (1951).

Eccles, J.C.: The brain-mind problem as a frontier of science. Progress in scientific culture, vol. 1, p. 1 (Bologna 1976).

Gastaut, H.; Tassinari, C.H.; Roger, J.; Soulayrol, R.; Saint Jean, M.; Regis, H.; Bernard, R.; Pinsard, N.; Dravet, C.: Juvenile epileptic encephalopathy associated with diffuse slow spike activity ('atypical petit mal', Lennox syndrome). Recenti Prog. Med. *45:* 117–146 (1968).

Giannitrapani, D.: EEG differences between resting and mental multiplication. Percept. Mot. Skills *22:* 399–405 (1966).

Giannitrapani, D.: EEG average frequency and intelligence. Electroenceph. clin. Neurophysiol. *27:* 480–486 (1969).

Giannitrapani, D.: Spectral analysis of the EEG; in Dolce, Künkel, CEAN, Computerized EEG analysis, pp. 384–402 (Fischer, Stuttgart 1975).

Giannitrapani, D.: Spatial organization of the EEG in normal and schizophrenic subjects. Electromyogr. clin. Neurophysiol. *19:* 125–145 (1979a).

Giannitrapani, D.: Laterality preference, electrophysiology and the brain. Electromyogr. clin. Neurophysiol. *19:* 105–123 (1979b).

Giannitrapani, D.; Bertrand, J.; Saucer, R.T.: Fourier analysis resolution of EEG frequency components of short duration. Electromyogr. clin. Neurophysiol. *23:* 613–626 (1983).

Giannitrapani, D.; Rast, V.T.; Shulhafer, B.J.: Computers in behavioral science: multiple channel direct digital recording of EEG data. Behav. Sci. *16:* 239–243 (1971).

Giannitrapani, D.; Sorkin, A.; Enenstein, J.: Laterality preference of children and adults as related to interhemispheric EEG phase activity. J. neurol. Sci. *3:* 139–151 (1966).

Giannitrapani, D.; Stoddard, V.: Frontal-lobes' role in thinking: EEG findings. Am. Psychol. *15:* 480 (1960).

Gibbs, E.L.; Rich, C.L.; Fois, A.; Gibbs, F.A.: Electroencephalographic study of mentally retarded persons. Am. J. ment. Defic. *65:* 236–247 (1960).

Gloor, P. (transl.; ed.): Hans Berger on the electroencephalogram of man. Electroenceph. clin. Neurophysiol., suppl. 28 (1969).

Hagberg, B.; Sjögren, I.: The sequelae of infantile hydrocephalus. Concours méd. *90:* 7055–7058 (1968).

Henry, C.E.: Electroencephalograms of normal children. Monograph of the Society for Research in Child Development, vol. XI (Natn. Research Council, Washington 1944).

Jenkins, C.D.: The relation of EEG slowing to selected indices of intellectual impairment. J. nerv. ment. Dis. *135:* 162–170 (1962).

Knott, J.R.; Friedman, H.; Bardsley, R.: Some electroencephalographic correlates of intelligence in eight-year- and twelve-year-old children. J. exp. Psychol. *30:* 380–391 (1942).

Kreezer, G.: Intelligence level and occipital alpha rhythm in the mongolian type of mental deficiency. Am. J. Psychol. *52:* 503–532 (1939).

Kreezer, G.; Smith, F.W.: The relation of the alpha rhythm of the electroencephalogram and intelligence level in the non-differentiated familial type of mental deficiency. J. Psychol. *29:* 47–51 (1950).

Liberson, W.T.: Ondes électriques du cerveau et intelligence; PhD thesis, Montréal (mimeographed, 1950).

Liberson, W.T.: Ondes électriques du cerveau et intelligence chez les malades mentaux. L'Année Psychologique, pp. 677–703 (Presses Universitaires de France, Paris 1951).

Liberson, W.T.: EEG and intelligence; in Zubin, Jarvik, Psychopathology of mental development, pp. 514–543 (Grune & Stratton, New York 1967).

Lindsley, D.B.: Electrical potentials of the brain in children and adults. J. gen. Psychol. *19:* 285–306 (1938).

Lindsley, D.B.: A longitudinal study of the occipital alpha rhythm in normal children: frequency and amplitude standards. J. genet. Psychol. *55:* 197–213 (1939).

Mundy-Castle, A.C.: Electrophysiological correlates of intelligence. J. Personality *26:* 184–199 (1958).

Netchine, S.; Lairy, G.C.: Ondes cérébrales et niveau mental: quelques aspects de l'évolution génétique du tracé EEG suivant le niveau mental. Enfance *4–5:* 427–439 (1960).

Netchine, S.; Lairy, G.C.: Comparison of EEG data and intelligence level in children; in Proc. London Conf. on the Scientific Study of Mental Deficiency, 1960, vol. 2, pp. 378–383 (May & Baker, Dagenham 1962).

Osaka, M.; Osaka, N.: Human intelligence and power spectral analysis of visual evoked potentials. Percept. Mot. Skills *50:* 192–194 (1980).

Saltzberg, B.; Burch, N.R.: A new approach to signal analysis in electroencephalography. IRE Trans. biomed. Engng *8:* 24–30 (1957).

Saltzberg, B.; Burch, N.R.: Period analytic estimates of moments of the power spectrum: a simplified EEG time domain procedure. Electroenceph. clin. Neurophysiol. *30:* 568–570 (1971).

Seppalainen, A.M.; Kivalo, E.: EEG findings and epilepsy in Down's syndrome. J. ment. Defic. Res. *11:* 116–125 (1967).

Shagass, C.: An attempt to correlate the occipital alpha frequency of the electroencephalogram with performance on a mental ability test. J. exp. Psychol. *36:* 88–92 (1946).

Shucard, D.W.; Horn, J.L.: Evoked cortical potentials and measurement of human abilities. J. comp. physiol. Psychol. *78:* 59–68 (1972).

Smith, J.R.: The electroencephalogram during normal infancy and childhood. II. The nature of the growth of the alpha waves. J. genet. Psychol. *53:* 455–469 (1938).

Smith, J.R.: The frequency growth of the human alpha rhythms during normal infancy and childhood. J. Psychol. *11:* 177–198 (1941).

Walter, D.O.; Rhodes, J.M.; Brown, D.; Adey, W.R.: Comprehensive spectral analysis of human EEG generators in posterior cerebral regions. Electroenceph. clin. Neurophysiol. *20:* 224–237 (1966).

Walter, W.G.: An improved low frequency analyser. Electron. Eng. *16:* 236–240 (1943).

Walters, C.: Clinical and experimental relationships of EEG to psychomotor and personality measures. J. clin. Psychol. *20:* 81–91 (1964).

Weinberg, H.: Correlation of frequency spectra of averaged visual evoked potentials with verbal intelligence. Nature, Lond. *224:* 813–815 (1969).

Werner, H.: Comparative psychology of mental development (Harper, New York 1940).

3 Samples, Tests, EEG-Spectral Analysis Considerations and Reliability Study

'The concept of a wave is perhaps the most profound in all of science. Wave propagation is nature's way of transmitting energy and information over long distances with a minimum of energy loss and little permanent distortion of the intervening medium.'
P.L. Nunez

Sample

One hundred 11- to 13-year-old residents of Oak Park, Illinois, constituted the sample pool. Subjects' variables studied were mental ability and laterality preference. To develop an adequate left preferent sample, an effort was made to seek out left-handed subjects. The incidence of left preference in this sample, therefore, is greater than its normal occurrence in a randomly selected population. Subjects were administered a Wechsler Intelligence Scale for Children (WISC) [*Wechsler,* 1949], 4 additional mental ability tests developed in our laboratory, a laterality preference test, and an EEG examination obtained during 8 behavioral states (cf. EEG Conditions).

From the pool of 100 subjects, samples were obtained as follows:

(1) All subjects for whom artifact-free EEG records were obtained (n = 83, all subjects of tables 3/I and 3/II) which included left, mixed and right-handed subjects. A limited number of correlations was performed for these data (reported in chapter 4) which were subsequently subdivided into separate samples according to the subjects' variables to be studied.

(2) 12 subjects for whom longitudinal data was obtained and analyzed for the reliability study (table 3/I, study 2, and the Reliability Study section in this chapter).

Table 3/I. Subjects' characteristics: study 1, all subjects (n = 83), chapter 4; study 2 (n = 12), reliability, cf. chapter 3; study 3 (n = 56), right-preferent sample, chapters 5, 7–13; study 4 (n = 20), left-preferent sample, chapter 6

Subjects				IQ scores			Studies		
No.	age	sex	lateral.	verbal	perform.	full	2	3	4
1	11–0	M	19	104	111	108	×	×	
2	11–0	M	17	121	92	108		×	
3	11–0	M	9	126	114	123			×
4	11–1	M	19	111	101	107		×	
5	11–1	M	20	148	139	148		×	
6	11–2	M	11	121	97	111			×
7	11–2	F	17	97	120	109		×	
8	11–2	M	19	103	110	107		×	
9	11–2	M	21	135	142	142	×	×	
10	11–3	M	17	104	117	111		×	
11	11–4	M	8	120	115	120			×
12	11–4	M	9	90	92	90			×
13	11–4	F	20	114	125	121		×	
14	11–4	M	12	104	111	108			×
15	11–5	M	18	75	90	80	×	×	
16	11–6	M	16	126	133	133		×	
17	11–6	F	18	94	86	89		×	
18	11–7	M	10	125	125	128			×
19	11–8	M	17	119	96	109	×	×	
20	11–8	M	20	100	124	112		×	
21	11–8	F	20	100	94	97		×	
22	11–8	F	19	109	114	112		×	
23	11–9	M	19	116	121	120		×	
24	11–9	M	16	90	101	95			
25	11–9	M	17	135	101	128		×	
26	11–9	F	17	101	138	120		×	
27	11–10	M	19	120	103	113		×	
28	11–10	M	10	142	125	137			×
29	11–11	M	21	104	108	107	×	×	
30	11–11	M	18	125	106	117		×	
31	11–11	M	17	110	104	108		×	
32	12–0	M	10	123	121	124			×
33	12–1	F	17	94	111	102		×	
34	12–1	M	18	133	114	126		×	
35	12–1	M	20	124	110	125		×	
36	12–2	M	20	104	114	109		×	
37	12–2	M	11	126	89	109			×
38	12–3	M	20	128	96	114	×	×	
39	12–3	M	9	130	122	129			×
40	12–3	F	18	114	108	112		×	
41	12–4	M	16	126	139	136			
42	12–4	M	21	109	133	123	×	×	
43	12–5	M	20	141	120	133	×	×	
44	12–5	M	21	125	94	111		×	
45	12–5	M	21	101	128	115		×	
46	12–5	M	21	97	125	112		×	
47	12–5	M	8	116	107	113			×
48	12–7	F	19	94	94	93		×	
49	12–7	F	18	111	114	114		×	
50	12–8	M	14	89	100	93			×

Table 3/I (cont.)

Subjects				IQ scores			Studies		
No.	age	sex	lateral.	verbal	perform.	full	2	3	4
51	12–8	M	19	139	127	131		×	
52	12–8	M	20	80	108	93		×	
53	12–9	M	10	125	113	121			×
54	12–10	M	20	116	111	115		×	
55	12–10	F	18	104	135	120		×	
56	12–11	M	17	123	90	108		×	
57	12–11	M	18	113	99	107	×	×	
58	12–11	M	16	99	74	85	×		
59	12–11	M	14	103	117	110			
60	12–11	M	18	110	115	114		×	
61	12–11	M	14	123	121	124			×
62	13–0	M	21	85	129	107		×	
63	13–0	M	15	100	96	98			
64	13–0	F	19	110	128	120		×	
65	13–0	F	20	111	87	100		×	
66	13–1	F	19	104	108	107		×	
67	13–2	M	11	80	92	84			×
68	13–2	M	11	94	85	88			×
69	13–3	M	14	142	108	128			
70	13–3	F	17	101	113	107		×	
71	13–4	M	16	125	118	124			
72	13–4	M	18	75	86	79	×	×	
73	13–4	M	19	85	100	91		×	
74	13–4	M	7	91	97	93			×
75	13–5	M	17	130	106	120		×	
76	13–5	M	8	110	106	109			×
77	13–6	F	18	147	132	144		×	
78	13–7	M	11	129	113	123			×
79	13–8	M	19	129	121	128		×	
80	13–9	M	13	142	127	138			×
81	13–10	F	17	104	100	102		×	
82	13–11	M	21	123	111	119	×	×	
83	13–11	F	20	84	76	78		×	

(3) All subjects (n = 56: 18 females and 38 males) who were right-preferent (as defined in the Laterality Preference section) and had an EEG free of gross artifacts were selected for the main body of this study for which correlations between EEG scores and intellectual variables and factor analyses were performed. Characteristics of the subjects of this sample are shown in tables 3/I and 3/II, study 3 (chapters 5, 7–13).

(4) 20 left-preferent subjects (correlation study) for whom a limited number of correlations between EEG and intellectual scores was performed (tables 3/I and 3/II, study 4, and chapter 6).

Table 3/II. Characteristics of distributions of age and IQ scores for the 3 subject groups (n = 83, n = 56, n = 20) for which correlations with EEG power scores were obtained

	Age	IQ scores		
		verbal	performance	full-scale
n = 83 (study 1)				
Lowest score	11–0	75	74	78
Highest score	13–11	148	142	148
Mean	12–4	112	110	113
Median	12–4	111	111	112
Sigma	0–10	17.4	15.2	15.2
Standard error of mean	0–1	1.9	1.7	1.7
n = 56 (study 3)				
Lowest score	11–0	75	76	78
Highest score	13–11	148	142	148
Mean	12–4	111	111	112
Median	12–3	110	111	112
Sigma	0–10	17.4	15.4	14.6
Standard error of mean	0–1	2.3	2.1	2.0
n = 20 (study 4)				
Lowest score	11–0	80	85	84
Highest score	13–9	142	127	138
Mean	12–4	115	109	113
Median	12–4	122	112	116
Sigma	0–11	18.0	13.2	16.4
Standard error of mean	0–2	4.0	3.0	3.7

Mental Ability Tests

The major test of intelligence employed in this study was the widely used WISC [*Wechsler,* 1949] which was administered and scored according to the standard instructions. In addition to the 10 subtests which constitute the core of the test, the optional Digit Span subtest was also administered routinely. In clinical practice this subtest of the verbal scale is often added at the option of the examiner. This subtest was also included in the battery for purposes of comparison with the Wechsler Adult Intelligence Scale [*Wechsler,* 1944]. As the WISC manual [1949] indicates, the Verbal Scale IQ was then prorated as per standard procedures. The weighted subtest scores as well as the 3 main IQ scores were used to correlate with the EEG scores.

In an attempt to tap intellectual functions seemingly not represented on the WISC, 4 additional intellectual tasks other than the WISC were also administered:

1. Spatial Relations. Taken from the US Employment Service's [1945] special aptitude tests, this is the 3-dimensional spatial relations test (CB-1-H). The required task is to recognize an object in 3 dimensions on the basis of a schematic drawing.

2. Symbol Manipulation. Developed in our laboratory, this test requires the subject to recognize the role of sequence in a series of alphabetical characters and to extrapolate from this sequence. A sample item is:

					(1)	(2)	(3)	(4)	(5)
aa	bb	cc	dd	....	a	b	c	d	e

and the correct answer is (5), the beginning of the next pair of characters. This test is grossly comparable to the abstraction test of the Shipley-Hartford scale [*Shipley,* 1940].

3. Verbal Analogies. This test was developed in our laboratory. A sample item is:

GREEN: GRASS;   BLUE: _____

in which the correct answer is 1 of 5 words offered in multiple choice.

4. Psychomotor Efficiency. The numbers comparison test (test I) of the Minnesota Vocational Test for Clerical Workers [1933]. The task is to identify as quickly as possible which pairs of multidigit numbers are identical.

Laterality Preference Test

To determine laterality preference, each subject was requested to perform 7 tasks: (1) handwriting; (2) reaching for an object; (3) quick draw of a gun; (4) aiming a rifle; (5) paper sighting; (6) kicking a ball, and (7) grip strength. Performance on each task was scored: 1 for left side response, 2 for intermediate or mixed reaction, and 3 for right side response. A high total score indicated right preference and a low total score left preference.

The 7 tasks were:

1. Handwriting. The subject was presented with a pad and pencil in the median plane and was asked to write his/her name. He/she was then required to write the name with the opposite hand. If, upon inspection, the 2 samples proved to be of the same quality, the performance on this task was scored intermediate, i.e. 2. Otherwise, the hand used in the first writing determined the score (1 for left and 3 for right).

2. Reaching for Object. The subject was presented with an object in the median plane and instructed to grasp it. The task was repeated for 4 different objects. A total of 3 or more left reaches was scored as 1; a total of 2 reaches of each hand was scored as 2; and a total of 3 or more right reaches was scored as 3.

3. Quick Draw of a Gun. The subject was requested to make a quick draw, western style, with an imaginary pistol. Two-gun draw (using both hands) was scored 2, and left and right draws were scored 1 and 3, respectively.

4. Aiming a Rifle. The subject was told to aim an imaginary rifle at the experimenter's nose. Performance was scored on the basis of shoulder, eye and trigger finger used. A completely left-sided aim was scored 1, a combination of left and right was scored 2 and a completely right-sided aim was scored 3.

5. Paper Sighting. While holding with both hands a sheet of paper with a 1-inch hole in the center, the subject was instructed to move the sheet toward his/her eyes 4 times without losing sight of a dot on another sheet of paper in the lap. If the subject sighted at least 3 times with the left eye, the score was 1; for 2 left and 2 right sightings, the subject received a score of 2; and for at least 3 sightings with the right eye the subject received a score of 3.

6. Kicking a Ball. The subject was presented with a ball on the floor directly in front of the feet and was asked to kick it. The task was repeated 4 times and scored as for the paper sighting task.

7. Grip Strength. The subject was asked to squeeze a dynamometer twice with each hand. Stronger grip in the left hand for both trials was scored 1; mixed trials was scored 2 and stronger grip in the right hand was scored 3.

The sum of the 7 measures provided a range of scores that was divided into 3 groups as follows: 7–11 for left preferents; 12–16 for mixed preferents; and 17–21 for right preferents.

EEG Montage and Recordings

EEG tracings were recorded simultaneously from 16 scalp areas (fig. 3/1). The location of electrodes was as follows: the temporal line conformed to the 10–20 system, and the 3 coronal planes (F_7–F_8, T_3–T_4, T_5–T_6) were trisected to generate 2 additional electrode placements each (fron-

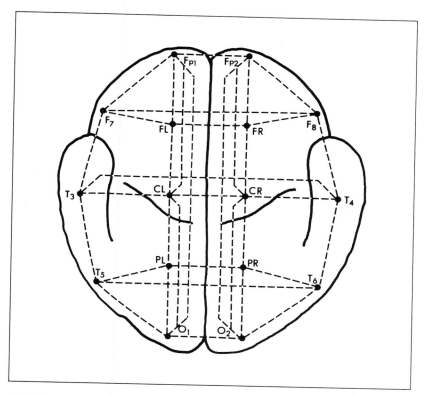

Fig. 3/1. Array of the 16 monopolar electrodes (combined ears used as reference) in which the temporal line conforms to the 10–20 system and the dashed lines refer to 36 interelectrode comparisons used for the cross-spectral determinations: Fp_1 Fp_2 = prefrontal left, right; F_7, F_8 = lateral frontal left, right; FL, FR = frontal left, right; CL, CR = central left, right; T_3, T_4 = temporal left, right; T_5, T_6 = post-temporal left, right; PL, PR = parietal left, right; O_1, O_2 = occipital left, right.

tal left and right or FL, FR, central left and right or CL, CR, and parietal left and right or PL, PR). This hybrid system was used in order to be able to record simultaneously from all scalp positions investigated. Given the hardware limitation of 16 EEG channels, the 10–20 system would have resulted in a nonequidistant placement of the median row of electrodes.

The method of recording was monopolar with combined ears as reference. While this preferential method assumes that the ears are silent, an assumption not always true, monopolar rather than bipolar recording was chosen because of the greater complexity of the rationale of bipolar recording when comparing findings of electrode pairs with noncommon references.

Gains of all preamplifiers were set at 0.5. Time constants of all preamplifiers were set at 0.3 s. Gains of all amplifiers were set at $\times$ 0.1, and gains of all postamplifiers were set at 100. In addition, the postamplifiers were finely tuned for equalization between channels.

The 16 channels of EEG were recorded on paper, and eight 8-second samples for each condition were concomitantly digitized and recorded on digital tape. Subsequently, one 8-second artifact-free record was selected for each of the 8 conditions for computer processing. Analysis consisted of Fourier analysis via computer program BMDX92 [*Massey and Jennrich*, 1969], i.e. spectral determinations from 0 to 34 Hz in 17 bands each 2-Hz wide for each of the 16 scalp areas tested.

Statistics reported related to 16 frequency bands from 2 to 34 Hz for data of the reliability study in this chapter and the data in chapters 4, 5 and 7, all based on 8 s of EEG. The main findings (chapters 8–13) were based on Spearman rhos computed for the 16 frequencies from 0 to 32 Hz based on 64 s of EEG. Data for the factor analysis of the EEG in chapter 15 was computed for 17 frequency bands from 0 to 34 Hz, also based on 64 s of EEG.

EEG Conditions and Analyses

In order to better evaluate the relationships with mental abilities, the EEG was obtained under a diverse array of behavioral states. It was hoped that spectral analysis was sensitive enough to discriminate not only between EEG activity occurring during auditory and visual modalities but also between different processing activities which would be present under different conditions within a given perceptual modality.

For the auditory modality it was felt desirable, if possible, to discriminate between 3 conditions: (1) unpatterned (white noise); (2) patterned nonverbal (music), and (3) patterned verbal (voice). If spectral analysis could accomplish this discrimination, the methodology could be used to study the distribution of EEG activity which related to higher cortical functions.

2 visual conditions were also adopted, 1 patterned (looking at a poster) and 1 unpatterned (looking through diffusing goggles). This would permit

partialing out changes due to visual stimulation and, in comparison with the noise condition, changes due to unpatterned stimulation. Other conditions consisted of performing mental arithmetic and of baseline awake resting at the beginning and end of the experiment.

Given the complexity of the experimental recording session, the 8 conditions were administered in the following order to all subjects:

(1) *Resting I* consisted of lying awake with eyes closed on a bed in a dark room for a period of 3 min.

(2) *Noise* (white noise), a sound source containing all frequencies in random distribution (e.g. FM radio noise between stations), consisted of listening to a white noise source of 50 dB for a period of 2 min.

(3) *Music* (listening to music), a 2-min excerpt from Tchaikovsky's *'Marche miniature'*.

(4) *Voice* (listerning to voice), a 2-min excerpt from Mark Twain's *Huckleberry Finn.*

(5) *Arithmetic* (mental arithmetic), silently performing mental arithmetic problems, i.e. mentally subtracting serial 7s from 100 and giving the answer aloud when reaching 0.

(6) *Vision* (patterned vision), looking at a geometric poster for 2 min.

(7) *Diffuse* (diffuse vision), looking through diffusing goggles, which permitted the subject to see only diffuse light, for 2 min.

(8) *Resting II* was the same as the first condition.

The basic analysis consisted of obtaining sets of correlations between each intellectual variable and the EEG power density estimates (17 frequency bands × 16 brain areas). Spearman rhos [*Siegel,* 1956] were chosen because of the absence of the linearity assumption. The correlations are presented in the form of matrices for each EEG condition or their average where the X axis displays the frequency bands (1–33) and the Y axis displays brain areas, each matrix displaying the correlations between the EEG scores and a single intellectual variable.

EEG Hardware

Conventional techniques utilized to obtain psychophysiological data suitable for computer analysis include direct and indirect methods whose effectiveness depends primarily on the kind of analysis desired and the quantity of data involved. A simple indirect method (off-line) may involve an individual's observing graphic records and copying amplitude and time measurements for key punching and presentation to the computer in card form. This method is impractical where detailed analysis is required and impossible where processing of large quantities of data is required.

The direct method (on-line) utilizes an analog-to-digital converter operating directly into the computer. This method was impractical at the time the data was collected due to the inefficient use of computer time and the difficulty for the computers available in 1966 to store large quantities of digitized data generated by 16 channels of multiples of 8-second time periods.

In the most commonly used off-line method the signals are recorded on magnetic tape using frequency modulation techniques. The data can then be reproduced for editing purposes and subsequent conversion to digital form. This method suffers from the fact that the FM technique introduces time and amplitudes errors which usually cannot be corrected in the analysis. Additional disadvantages are that analog tape is limited in the number of channels which can be recorded and that the subsequent digital conversion requires time-consuming procedures which increase the probablity of additional errors, both human and technical.

The system used in this study was designed to overcome the various disadvantages discussed. This system allows for recording of EEG or other psychophysiological data directly on digital computer tape at the time of data acquisition. Selected portions of the digital tape can then be processed in a large computer at a later date.

This system was designed to study the time-amplitude relationships of signals from the various brain areas through analysis of phase angle which had proven to be useful [*Giannitrapani,* 1965] and of Fourier transform and coherence [*Walter,* 1968].

Figure 3/2 shows the system in block diagram form and indicates the function performed by each basic component [*Giannitrapani* et al., 1971]. The signals are derived from traditional EEG components consisting of a Beckman Type R Oscillograph system. This unit includes 16 channels of preamplifiers and 17 power amplifiers. A 12-channel writer console was modified to accommodate 17 pen galvanometer units and 2 event markers. 16 pens were used to graphically record the 16 input signals while the 17th pen was used to monitor the digitizing process as explained later (fig. 3/3).

Signals for digital analysis were taken from the output of the preamplifiers through Beckman Type 428 postamplifiers. The use of these amplifiers allows independent adjustment and calibration of the signal being digitized and the pen galvanometer units.

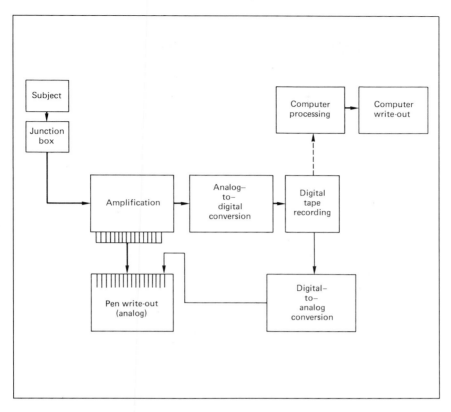

Fig. 3/2. Block diagram of the data acquisition system used in this study. From *Giannitrapani* et al. [1971], with permission *(Behavioral Science).*

After amplification and impedance matching, the signals were presented to the input of a combination multiplexer (signal scanner) and high speed analog-to-digital (A-to-D) converter manufactured from Raytheon components. Through a buffer this unit sequentially scans each input channel and converts the analog signal amplitude to a 12-bit binary word. The binary information is subsequently recorded on computer-compatible digital 0.5-inch magnetic tape by a recorder manufactured by Precision Instruments, Inc.

The entire system is controlled by a digital logic system designed and manufactured by Pivan Engineering Company, Chicago, Illinois. This controller is designed to provide a variety of automatic functions along with manual controls required for versatile operation of the system. The controller has provisions for determining the number of channels to be digitized, for regulating the number of scans per computer record (block), for determining the number of consecutive records and for identifying each record.

A 16-position switch selects the number of channels to be scanned (1–16). This switch, along with a crystal clock, determines the conversion rate (samples per second) for the selected channels. Since 16 channels were scanned, the system produces 128 samples/s for each of the channels.

The length of the computer record is determined by the number of scans via a set of 12 binary coded switches for any number of scans up to 4,096. For this research, the switches were set at 1,024, yielding a record of the duration of 8 s. The system permits recording up to 10 records sequentially with a thumbwheel switch with positions 0–9. Eight consecutive records were obtained in this investigation.

The control assembly includes a programming plug for use in determining the desired tape format (arrangement of the data on tape). The system is presently wired to record each 12-bit binary word as 2 subsequent 6-bit characters on the tape. This is accomplished by a shift register which delays one half of each conversion for appropriate character spacing.

A necessary capability of such a system is an automatic recording of 'heading information' which is placed at the beginning of each record for identification of the record in question. The system permits the recording on tape of 4 decimal digits as the first 4 characters of each record as determined by 4 external thumbwheel switches. The first 2 are used as subject identification numbers; the third is used as the experimental condition number; and the fourth determines the number of records to be recorded as mentioned earlier. It has an automatic step-up feature whereby the fourth character of each subsequent record is identified with consecutive digits (0–9) up to the digit present in the external thumbwheel switch.

This identification method has proved invaluable for obtaining inventories of records on a given tape and for guaranteeing that the record requested for a given analysis was the one that was actually analyzed. The channels are automatically identified by the fact that following the heading information, the scans always begin with channel 1 and proceed sequentially. The identification procedure, however, has not been entirely trouble-free because the heading information is recorded in binary-coded-decimal format while the data is recorded in binary 2s complement form. The mixed

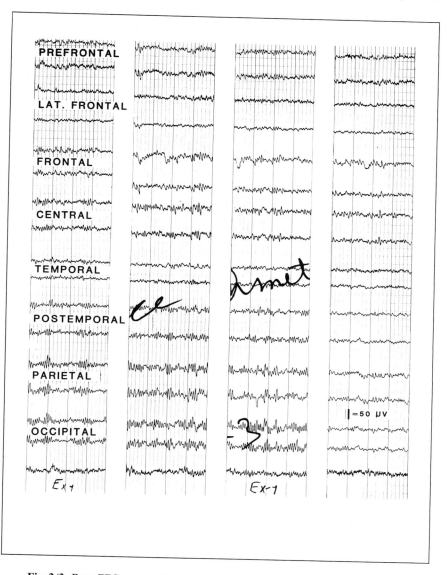

Fig. 3/3. Raw EEG record showing 4-second excerpts from subject No. 16 for the Resting I, Music, Arithmetic and Diffuse vision conditions. Note the difficulty in visually discriminating between the conditions. All odd-numbered channels are on the left side, even-numbered channels on the right. The 17th channel is monitoring (reversed polarity) the first channel (prefrontal left), and it consists of the reconstituted digital signal read from the tape.

mode thus obtained (all with negative parity) required machine language programming.

An additional provision of this system is the capability of reconstructing the data from any one of the channels to its original analog form. This is accomplished by a single-channel digital-to-analog converter. A 16-position switch provides selection of the channel to be reconstructed and recorded by the 17th pen of the console. This playback process is available in the read mode of the tape recorder but, even more important, it is available as an on-line monitoring device. In other words, during the digitizing and recording process, any one of the channels can be monitored through an analog playback of the reconstituted signal (fig. 3/3).

This provision is extremely valuable because it insures that the signals are actually being recorded and also because it facilitates the calibration routine. With the AC couplers there are known DC baseline interchannel differences that can be quickly monitored and equalized by manually scanning the 16-position switch and adjusting the zero levels. In this manner all channels are maintained within the sensitivity range of the digitizer without distortions due to electronic 'limiting'.

The research discussed here was performed by obtaining the EEG with traditional amplification and recording methods and, in addition, by recording on-line the EEG signals in digital form on computer tape. The digitized signals were processed off-line in a large computer to obtain auto-spectra, cross-spectra, phase-angle and coherence values. These, in turn, were stored on digital tape or in punched card form for later statistical analysis.

A basic advantage of on-line A-to-D conversion is the capability of storing 16 concomitant channels of EEG in a form that, when repeatedly retrieved for numerical analysis, is not subject to change. Central to the system is an A-to-D converter of great reliability and with a resolution surpassing the expected accuracy needs of the investigations.

One of the main advantages of computerized EEG analysis is the possibility that all the needed information may be extracted from extremely short samples. For this study a method was used which preserves the entire EEG record in its traditional ink-paper form so that it is available for comparison with the sections which have been processed in the computer.

Manual record identification at the time of recording permits accurate retrieval. Accuracy is guaranteed by maintaining, at the time of recording, a logbook identifying by number and function the EEG sections digitized and recorded on tape.

Sampling Rate

One of the first considerations when converting data from analog to digital form is the sampling rate or the number of measurements taken of the analog signal each second in time. The lower limit is given by the mathematical constraints requiring a sampling rate twice the fastest frequency to be studied (Nyquist frequency). To reconstitute a signal obtained by a standard EEG polygraph with characteristic rapid amplitude falloff beyond 30 Hz, a sampling rate of 60 Hz can be reconstituted in its analog form with traditional paper amplitude and speed without visible loss.

There is a problem in the a priori choice: if the purpose is to reproduce current EEG ink tracings with current fidelity, a sampling rate of 60 Hz is adequate, as mentioned above, but if investigations are being carried out for the purpose of determining what new findings can be obtained, then the choice is not so simple. While *Bremer* [1944] reported having observed EEG activity above 100 Hz and *Trabka* [1962] over 200 Hz, the increase of the number of conversions necessary for studying an unknown frequency range may create staggering computational problems.

Traditional EEG analysis terminated in the 30-Hz range for basically two reasons: (1) in and above that range EEG was undistinguishable from muscle artifact, and (2) at 60 Hz there were serious problems of interference with power line oscillations which the old amplifiers had difficulty in isolating. With solid-state electronics the 60-Hz interference has been reduced considerably and can be reduced even further if valuable information found in that frequency range should require it. If valuable information is found between 25 and 60 Hz, computerized EEG analysis methods can be developed to partial out muscle artifacts by appropriate patterning, triangulation and statistial analyses.

The present investigations were concerned with EEG steady states rather than short transients. Given certain computer storage constraints and computer program limits, the length of the period that can be analyzed is inversely related to the sampling rate. It was considered desirable to be able to analyze the traditional EEG range plus a few additional faster frequencies for exploration purposes.

The sampling rate of 128 conversions/s was arrived at through consideration of the following. One of the first aims of the project was to demonstrate that digitization and computer analysis of the EEG did permit the observation of already known EEG phenomena. The study of 0–30 Hz was therefore mandatory. To resolve the fastest frequency component in this range by digital techniques, the quoted Nyquist frequency is 60 Hz.

The effective sampling rate figure should be doubled since numerical prefiltering with a decimation ratio of 2 was used. The sampling rate therefore was 128 conversions/s, a power of 2 which permitted a certain ease in programming [*Massey and Jennrich,* 1969]. Numerical prefiltering is highly desirable for eliminating those higher frequencies present in the raw tracing which would be reflected in the frequency range studied, introducing an error in the measurements.

Resolution of A-to-D Conversion

The voltage resolution or accuracy of an A-to-D conversion unit adequate for EEG recording is usually quoted in 'bits' which have to be translated into microvolts to be meaningful to the electroencephalographer.

A resolution of 1 μV, which is less than the pen tracing width in a traditional EEG record, would permit reconstituting the analog tracing without visible loss in amplitude differentials. The research problems, however, are similar to those which occur in arriving at the determination of the sampling rate. Barring signal-to-noise ratio limitations, with computerized EEG analysis methods it should be possible to obtain findings related to amplitude differentials unobservable in the traditional recording.

The Multiverter chosen for the A-to-D conversion has a 12-bit resolution which means that it discriminates 1 part in 4,096. In common EEG voltage terminology, this means that at a standard gain setting the EEG voltage range acceptable to the system is in steps of 0.122 μV for a total range of 500 μV. This degree of accuracy seems excessive to one accustomed to visually analyzing ink-paper records in which the ink tracing is broader than 1 μV.

To avoid changing amplifier gains during recordings (a valuable consideration for a signal which is stored numerically in a nonimmediately visible form), a range of 500 μV is believed to be adequate to record even high-voltage transients, such as paroxysmal discharges, with little limiting effect. The increase in accuracy and the broad range of response provide greater reliability of the Fourier analysis on one hand and better control of the interchannel DC level differences on the other.

The system is confronted with 3 oscillating frequencies extraneous to the signal. They are the frequency of the vibrators of the preamps at 400 Hz, the A-to-D conversion frequency of 128 Hz, and the line current of 60 Hz. The harmonics of these frequencies interacting in the range of 0–32 Hz are: (1) a beat frequency produced by the third harmonic of 128 Hz, and (2) the fundamental of 400 Hz which occurs at 16 Hz and a beat frequency produced by the second harmonic of the 60 Hz and the fundamental of 128 Hz which occurs at 8 Hz near the alpha activity band. The occurrence of amplitude peaks at these frequencies needs to be interpreted guardedly.

Length of the Sample

Some of the ideas concerning traditional EEG recording need to be modified when utilizing computerized EEG analysis. One of these concerns the EEG record length. The procedure used at this laboratory required for each condition the routine analysis of one or two 8-second periods of EEG, but to allow for elimination of periods containing artifacts, 8 such periods were recorded consecutively. Each period was referred to as a computer record. Recording was decided upon by observing the occurrence of an artifact-free section for a given condition and then pushing the recording button with the expectation that this artifact-free section would continue.

It is necessary to make an a priori choice of accumulating data of a certain sample-length in the expectation of developing fruitful correlates unless one uses a continuous recording method [*Petsche,* 1967; *Shaw,* 1970]. The body of knowledge stems primarily from naturalistic observation of the tracings with the conclusion that EEG states fluctuate at rates anywhere from a fraction of a second upward. Computerized EEG analysis, however, had its forerunner in electronic frequency analysis with the work of *Baldock and Walter* [1946] which demonstrated a certain amplitude similarity in subsequent 10-second epochs. Particular emphasis to amplitude analysis has recently been given by *Goldstein* [1975, 1983] in the tradition of *Liberson* [1936] and *Drohocki* [1937, 1969]. *Goldstein* accomplished the amplitude analysis by integrating EEG signals from different brain areas with a bank of solid-state integrators. He has utilized this technique in studying characteristics from psychopharmacology [*Goldstein* et al., 1965], hemispheric asymmetries [*Goldstein* et al., 1972], psychopathology [*Goldstein and Stoltzfus,* 1973] and behavioral traits and states [*Goldstein,* 1983].

Electroencephalographers have shunned studies of EEG variability probably because of the difficulty in quantifying EEG signals prior to the availability of computers and the difficulties in defining criterion variables (e.g. behavioral states). Notable exceptions are the work of *Davis* [1940], *Sugerman* et al. [1964] with schizophrenics, *Goldstein* et al. [1963] and *Goldstein and Stoltzfus* [1973] with drugs and *Goldstein* et al. [1970] for sleep. The study of EEG variability per se was performed by *Remond* [1956], *Byford* [1965], *Matoušek and Volavka* [1965], *Künkel* et al. [1969], *Giannitrapani* [1975] and *Giannitrapani and Roccaforte* [1975].

Interchannel Discrepancies

A relatively unexplored difficulty in computerized EEG analysis has been the problem of discrepancies in the behavior of supposedly identical amplifiers. Considerable differences were observed among the spectral density values obtained from the output of different channels from a common EEG input. This occurred after normal calibration within the tolerances normally used for visual scoring. Replacement and matching capacitors with 1% tolerance and peaking of the amplifiers with precise electronic procedures did not suffice to eliminate the problem which was placing severe limitations on the reliability of digital techniques.

The pre-and postamplifiers were calibrated so that with an input of 50 μV at 10 Hz, a signal level of 2 V (± 0.1) peak-to-peak was entered into the Multiverter. The single-channel digital-to-analog converter was then employed to verify that when a common signal was recorded on all 16 channels, the wave forms recovered from its digital representations would, in fact, look like the original signal. With the equipment thus calibrated, the signal from an occipital lead was entered into all 16 channels simultaneously, and 8 second records were digitized for spectral analysis (the advantage of using the EEG in place of an artificially produced calibration signal is that the EEG contains all the various frequency components at roughly the intensity in which they will be encountered during actual recording and thus provides a more realistic test of the apparatus).

As mentioned earlier, considerable disagreement among the spectral measurements from different channels was found originally. Not only was the power density of a given frequency band different for each of the 16 amplifiers, but the ratios of spectral densities from corresponding frequency bands for a single pair of amplifiers varied substantially across frequencies. These variations are attributable to 3 factors: (1) differences in gain adjustment between amplifiers, (2) a small but measurable drift in the postamplifier gains, and (3) discrepancies in the RC characteristics of the coupler circuitry of the preamplifiers.

2 methods, 1 electronic and 1 numerical, were introduced to deal with the problem. The electronic method consisted of recording twice, consecutively, the data from a given condition with 2 different montages between electrodes and amplifiers so that a particular activity observed in the output of a given channel could be checked on a later date to determine whether it originated in the electronic equipment or in the brain.

The numerical method consisted of an elaborate routine to normalize all data against correction factors derived from the average of 2 sets of spectral density values obtained from a common EEG input to all 16 channels. 1 set was at the beginning and 1 set at the end of each experimental run [*Clusin* et al., 1970]. Separate correction coefficients were determined for each frequency band for each channel. Thus, 272 different coefficients (16 brain areas × 17 frequency bands) were used to normalize each run.

Analysis of the 2 methods demonstrated the superiority of the numerical method and the superfluousness of the electronic method. The numerical routine is excellent in eliminating interchannel discrepancies, and the correction coefficients obtained can be inspected to determine the magnitude of the errors in the system and when certain electronic components need to be replaced.

Reliability Study

To determine the degree of reliability of different sample lengths, the following analysis was performed. The digitized EEGs of 12 male right-preferent 11- to 13-year-old subjects selected from our subject pool were subjected to Fourier analysis from 2 to 34 Hz in 16 bands, 2 Hz wide for each of 16 brain areas recorded concomitantly.

One of the purposes of the investigation was to study the possibly different reliabilities of different frequency bands in different brain areas, hence the variables mentioned above. Interacting with these variables was the possibility of changes in reliability of a given sample length depending on different behavioral states. Hence the EEG was studied under the 8 conditions of this study (cf. EEG Conditions).

Reliability of sample lengths was to be determined through Pearson r^2 values representing variances or percentage of agreement between the 2 samples. Sample lengths used were 8, 16 and 32 s, while time intervals

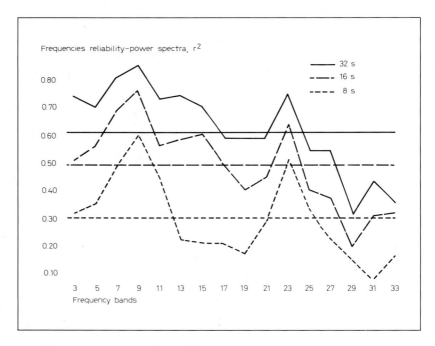

Fig. 3/4. Autospectra reliability of different EEG frequencies (brain areas pooled) for records of 8, 16 and 32 s duration of the resting condition with an inter-record distance of 40 min. Horizontal lines represent the mean reliability of each record length. From *Giannitrapani* [1975], with permission (Fischer, Stuttgart).

between samples were approximately 10, 40 s, and 40 min. A repeated measurement factorial-design analysis of variance was performed on the r^2 values of the autospectral data described.

Data show, in samples 40 min apart, an average 30% agreement between 8-second samples and an average 62% agreement between 32-second samples. The distribution of scores indicates small increments with decreasing intersample distances but larger increments with increasing sample length.

These averages, however, are not informative of the reliability of individual frequencies nor of individual brain areas. An indication of this is shown in figure 3/4 which expands for frequencies the figures quoted above for autospectra and in figure 3/5 which expands the same data, showing instead separate values for the different brain areas.

The degree of parallelism of the 3 lines in each graph indicates that

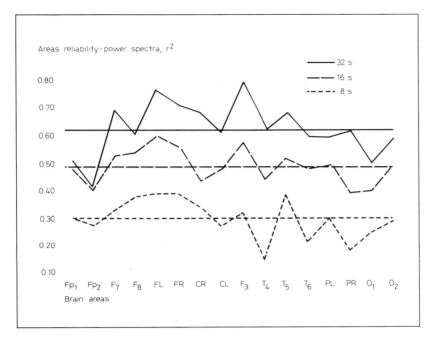

Fig. 3/5. Autospectra reliability containing the same data as figure 3/3 but showing the mean values for the 16 brain areas studied (frequencies pooled). From *Giannitrapani* [1975], with permission (Fischer, Stuttgart).

even in the 8-second sample, while reliability is lower, it is nevertheless representative of the features of longer sample lengths. In this shortest time period with an average of r^2 of 0.30, r^2 of individual frequencies are as high as 0.60 for the 9-Hz band (not dominant alpha which for this group is in the 11-Hz band) and 0.51 for the 23-Hz activity which will be shown in this study to be particularly related to intellectual functioning.

Figure 3/5, showing the reliability of EEG frequencies in different brain areas, indicates that most areas in the left hemisphere have a larger percentage of agreement than those in the right hemisphere (all odd-numbered electrodes are placed on the left hemisphere), a finding of consequence considering that all 12 subjects of this study were right-preferents. This is an example of findings by serendipity in which, while studying EEG sample lengths, one can uncover what could be a major finding concerning the higher reliability of the activity of the dominant hemisphere.

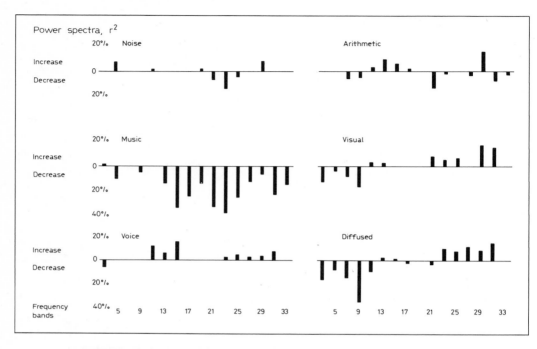

Fig. 3/6. Increase and decrease in reliability between resting and the stimulus conditions (expressed in %). The reliabilities between two 16-second records with a 40-second interval for each of the 6 stimulus conditions were compared with the reliabilities of the 2 resting conditions (of comparable length and inter-record intervals), separately for each frequency band, brain areas pooled. From *Giannitrapani* [1975], with permission (Fischer, Stuttgart).

Reliability varied also depending on the behavioral state of the subject while the EEG was recorded. The 6 stimulus conditions of the study were utilized (cf. EEG Conditions). Figure 3/6 shows changes in r^2 between these conditions and the extreme of the 2 resting r^2, the latter being represented as a straight line. A line extending upward indicates an increase and downward a decrease in the reliability between two 16-second periods of a given condition recorded with a 40-second interval when compared with the reliability of either of the 2 resting conditions. The figure shows the greatest decrease in reliability occurring while listening to music. The greatest increase in reliability was in the dominant alpha band while listening to a story and in the beta frequencies during the eyes-open conditions.

References

Baldock, G.R.; Walter, W.G.: A new electronic analyzer. Electron. Eng. *18:* 339–342 (1946).

Bremer, F.: L'activité 'spontanée' des centres nerveux. Bull. Acad. méd. Belg. *11:* 148–173 (1944).

Byford, G.H.: Signal variance and its application to continuous measurements of EEG activity. Proc. R. Soc. *161:* 421–437 (1965).

Clusin, W.; Giannitrapani, D.; Roccaforte, P.: A numerical approach to matching amplification for the spectral analysis of recorded EEG. Electroenceph. clin. Neurophysiol. *28:* 639–641 (1970).

Davis, P.A.: Evaluation of the electroencephalogram of schizophrenic patients. Am. J. Psychiat. *96:* 851–860 (1940).

Drohocki, Z.: Die spontane elektrische Spannungsproduktion der Grosshirnrinde. Pflügers Arch. ges. Physiol. *239:* 658–679 (1937).

Drohocki, Z.: L'utilisation d'un analyseur statistique d'amplitudes, ASA, en électroencéphalographie quantitative. J. Physiol., Paris *61:* suppl. 2, part 2 (Communications), p. 275 (1969).

Giannitrapani, D.: EEG phase asymmetries and laterality preference. Clin. Neurophysiol. EEG-EMG Commun., pp. 301–305 (Vienna Medical Academy, Vienna 1965).

Giannitrapani, D.: Spectral analysis of the EEG; in Dolce, Künkel, CEAN, computerized EEG analysis, pp. 384–402 (Fischer, Stuttgart 1975).

Giannitrapani, D.; Rast, V.T.; Shulhafer, B.J.: Computers in behavioral science: multiple channel direct digital recording of EEG data. Behav. Sci. *16:* 239–243 (1971).

Giannitrapani, D.; Roccaforte, P.: Reliability measurements of EEG components in different behavioral states; in Matejcek, Schenk, Quantitative analysis of the EEG. Proc. 2nd Symp. Study Group for EEG Methodology, Jongny-sur-Vevey 1975, pp. 761–772.

Goldstein, L.: Time domain analysis of the EEG. The integrative method; in Dolce, Künkel, CEAN, computerized EEG analysis, pp. 251–270 (Fischer, Stuttgart 1975).

Goldstein, L.: Some EEG correlates of behavioral traits and states in humans. Res. Commun. psychol. psychiat. Behav. *8:* 115–142 (1983).

Goldstein, L.; Burdick, J.A.; Laszlo, M.: A quantitative analysis of the EEG during sleep in normal subjects. Acta physiol. hung. *37:* 291–300 (1970).

Goldstein, L.; Murphree, H.B.; Sugerman, A.A.; Pfeiffer, C.C.; Jenney, E.H.: Quantitative electroencephalographic analysis of naturally occurring (schizophrenic) and drug-induced psychotic states in human males. Clin. Pharmacol. Ther. *4:* 10–21 (1963).

Goldstein, L.; Stoltzfus, N.M.: Psychoactive drug-induced changes of interhemispheric EEG amplitude relationships. Agents Actions *3:* 124–132 (1973).

Goldstein, L.; Stoltzfus, N.M.; Gardocki, J.F.: Changes in interhemispheric amplitude relationships in the EEG during sleep. Physiol. Behav. *8:* 811–815 (1972).

Goldstein, L.; Sugerman, A.A.; Stolberg, H.; Murphree, H.B.; Pfeiffer, C.C.: Electrocerebral activity in schizophrenic and non-psychotic subjects: quantitative EEG amplitude analysis. Electroenceph. clin. Neurophysiol. *19:* 350–361 (1965).

Künkel, H.; Schweitzer, F.; Sternberg, M.; Sternberg, P.: Power spectral analysis of higher central nervous rhythms in the human EEG. Electroenceph. clin. Neurophysiol. *27:* 677 (1969).

Liberson, W.T.: Electroencéphalographie transcrânienne chez l'homme. Travail hum. *4:* 303–320 (1936).

Massey, F., III; Jennrich, R.: BMDX92: time series spectrum estimation; in Dixon, BMD biomedical computer programs, X series, pp. 193–224 (University of California Press, Berkeley 1969).

Matoušek, M.; Volavka, J.: Variability – an important dimension of EEG. Clin. Neurophysiol. EEG-EMG Commun., pp. 559–562 (Vienna Medical Academy, Vienna 1965).

Minnesota Vocational Test for Clerical Workers. (Psychological Corp., New York 1933).

Petsche, H.: Die Erfassung von Form und Verhalten der Potentialfelder an der Hirnoberfläche durch eine kombinierte EEG-toposkopische Methode. Wien. Z. NervHeilk. *25:* 373–387 (1967).

Remond, A.: Intégration temporelle et spatiale à l'aide d'un même appareil. Revue neurol. *95:* 585–586 (1956).

Shaw, J.C.: A method for continuously recording characteristics of EEG topography. Electroenceph. clin. Neurophysiol. *29:* 592–601 (1970).

Shipley, W.C.: A self-administering scale for measuring intellectual impairment and deterioration. J. Psychol. *9:* 371–377 (1940).

Siegel, S.: Nonparametric statistics for the behavioral sciences (McGraw-Hill, New York 1956).

Sugerman, A.; Goldstein, L.; Murphree, H.; Pfeiffer, C.; Jenney, E.: EEG and behavioral changes in schizophrenia: a quantitative study. Archs gen. Psychiat. *10:* 340–344 (1964).

Trabka, J.: High frequency components in brain wave activity. Electroenceph. clin. Neurophysiol. *14:* 453–464 (1962).

US Employment Service: Test CB-1-H (Occupational Analysis and Industrial Services Div., Dept. of Labor, Washington 1945).

Walter, D.O.: Coherence as a measure of relationship between EEG recordings. Electroenceph. clin. Neurophysiol. *24:* 282P (1968).

Wechsler, D.: The measurement of adult intelligence; 3rd ed. (Williams & Wilkins, Baltimore 1944).

Wechsler, D.: WISC manual, Wechsler Intelligence Scale for Children (Psychological Corp., New York 1949).

II First Correlation Matrices

'I was never happy about a definition of the alpha rhythm for I don't think it is a single process at all.'
W. Grey Walter

4 Auto- and Cross-Spectra of the Full Subjects' Sample

'... imaginary numbers ... are a wonderful flight of God's spirit.'
Leibnitz on complex numbers

Early analysis of the data includes 4 sets of correlational analyses. The first 2 sets were performed on the full subject sample of n = 83 on auto-spectral data of 3 conditions (tables 4/I–4/V) and on autospectral and cross-spectral data of the mental Arithmetic condition (fig. 4/1–4/5). The second 2 corresponding sets, performed on the right-handed portion of the sample (n = 56) on autospectral data of 3 conditions (tables 5/I–5/III) and on auto- and cross-spectral data of the mental Arithmetic condition (fig. 5/1–5/5), will be discussed in chapter 5. The range of frequencies for which rhos were computed for both chapters was from 2 to 34 Hz in 16 bands each 2-Hz wide.

From the pool of 100 subjects, all subjects for whom artifact-free EEG records were obtained constituted a group of 83 which included left-handed, mixed, and right-handed subjects. The first analyses were performed on this sample for each of the 8 conditions separately. The spectrum of 8 s of EEG was analyzed for each subject, and these autospectral values were correlated via Spearman rhos with each subtest score and IQ scores of the Wechsler Intelligence Scale for Children (WISC) [*Wechsler*, 1949]. Of the almost 30,000 Spearman rho values obtained for this first autospectral analysis, the occurrence of values significant at the 0.05, 0.01 and 0.001 levels by far exceed chance expectation. Since isolated values, even though significant, may occur by chance in such a large matrix of correlations, isolated findings are ignored and discussion is restricted to the clusters of patterning of significant rhos. Only selected data from 3 conditions is discussed in the first set of analyses.

Table 4/I shows 3 matrices of significant rhos obtained between 8 s of EEG acquired during 3 conditions: Resting I, mental Arithmetic and Resting II, when correlated with scores of the WISC coding subtest which requires efficient visual tracking, a certain amount of memory and visual motor performance. To permit better readability, these matrices show only rhos significant beyond the 0.05 level. All 3 conditions show a cluster of significant positive correlations in the occipital areas. The mental Arithmetic condition shows a cluster of significant negative correlations in the anterior areas in a slow frequency band where the power of eye-movement artifact occurs. Some subjects' involuntary eye movements are known to increase during mental Arithmetic. A possible reason for the negative rhos is that Coding requires efficient and speedy eye movement between the code and the target, and it is quite possible that the subject who has involuntary eye movements during mental Arithmetic finds it difficult to engage in volitional eye movements with speed and precision and will consequently be penalized in this timed visual task.

If the above-mentioned rationale is correct, it has been found by serendipity that the subject with involuntary eye movements during mental Arithmetic has a visuo-motor system which is not easily brought under voluntary control.

The matrix of rhos between EEG frequencies and the WISC Coding subtest is among those with the fewest significant correlations. The subtest with the most significant correlations is Comprehension. The same EEG scores used in table 4/I are correlated in table 4/II with the corresponding WISC Comprehension weighted scores. The striking characteristics of this table are again the degree of the reproducibility of 8 s of EEG under different conditions and the fact that many brain areas and many frequencies are involved with little or no relationship being shown in the occipital areas which were prominent in the Coding subtest. In terms of frequencies, the 11-Hz band (which includes the dominant alpha frequency for the sample) shows a moderate amount of relationship and not in the occipital areas (where the amplitude of dominant activity is the highest). The strongest relationships are found in the 13-Hz band instead, a frequency band which has an amplitude many times smaller than that of 11-Hz activity. In the higher frequencies, there is a notable cluster of significant relationships in the anterior areas for the 23-Hz band. It is relevant to note that this particular frequency was among the highest in the reliability of its amplitude scores (fig. 3/3) [*Giannitrapani and Roccaforte*, 1975] while the reliability of the 13-Hz activity for its second period is lower than in all the slower frequencies.

Table 4/I. WISC Coding vs 8 s of EEG power (autospectra) for 3 conditions: Resting I, mental Arithmetic and Resting II for all subjects (n = 83), significant rhos

		Frequency bands															
		3	5	7	9	11	13	15	17	19	21	23	25	27	29	31	33
Resting I																	
Prefrontal	left																
	right																
Lat. frontal	left																
	right																
Frontal	left																
	right																
Central	left																
	right																
Temporal	left																
	right																
Post-temporal	left																
	right																
Parietal	left																
	right																
Occipital	left										•	•						
	right						•			•	●						•	
Mental Arithmetic																	
Prefrontal	left																
	right	−•															
Lat. frontal	left																
	right	−•															
Frontal	left	−•	−•														
	right	−•															•
Central	left												•				
	right																
Temporal	left																
	right																
Post-temporal	left																
	right															•	
Parietal	left																
	right											•					
Occipital	left											•	●	•			
	right									•	•	●	•			•	
Resting II																	
Prefrontal	left																
	right																
Lat. frontal	left																
	right																
Frontal	left	−•															
	right																
Central	left																
	right																
Temporal	left																
	right																
Post-temporal	left																
	right																
Parietal	left																
	right																
Occipital	left						•										
	right						•		•	•		•	•				

• Rho with $p < 0.05$ (0.22–0.27); ● rho with $p < 0.01$ (0.28–0.35); ● rho with $p < 0.001$ (0.36–0.42); ■ rho with $p < 0.0001$ (> 0.42).
A minus (−) preceding the dot indicates a negative rho.

Table 4/II. WISC Comprehension vs 8 s of EEG power (autospectra) for 3 conditions: Resting I, mental Arithmetic and Resting II for all subjects (n = 83), significant rhos

		3	5	7	9	11	13	15	17	19	21	23	25	27	29	31	33
		\multicolumn{16}{Frequency bands}

Resting I

		3	5	7	9	11	13	15	17	19	21	23	25	27	29	31	33
Prefrontal	left											•					
	right																
Lat. frontal	left						•			•		●					
	right						•										
Frontal	left				•		•				•	•	•				
	right				•												
Central	left						●										
	right					•	•										
Temporal	left						•			•							
	right		•				•										
Post-temporal	left																
	right																
Parietal	left																
	right																
Occipital	left																
	right																

Mental Arithmetic

		3	5	7	9	11	13	15	17	19	21	23	25	27	29	31	33
Prefrontal	left						•					•					
	right																
Lat. frontal	left		•	•			●	•				●					
	right							•				•					
Frontal	left			•			●	•				●					
	right		•	●			●	●				●					
Central	left	•	•	●			●	•				•					
	right			●			●					●		•			
Temporal	left	•	•	•			●										
	right	•	•	•													
Post-temporal	left						•										
	right			•													
Parietal	left		•				•								•		
	right																
Occipital	left																
	right																

Resting II

		3	5	7	9	11	13	15	17	19	21	23	25	27	29	31	33
Prefrontal	left																
	right						•	•									
Lat. frontal	left	•	●	•		•	●	•				●	•				
	right		●			•						•					
Frontal	left		●	•			•	•				•	•				
	right		■	●	•	•	●	●	•	•	●	●	•				
Central	left	●	●		•		●	●									
	right	●	●	•		•	●	•				•					
Temporal	left	●	●	●	•	•	●	•									
	right		●			•	●										
Post-temporal	left	•	●	•			●	•				•					
	right	●	●	●			●										
Parietal	left	●	■	●			●	●				●					
	right	●	●	●			●	●				•					
Occipital	left	•	●														
	right	●	●	•			•										

• Rho with p < 0.05 (0.22–0.27); ● rho with p < 0.01 (0.28–0.35); ● rho with p < 0.001 (0.36–0.42); ■ rho with p < 0.0001 (> 0.42).
A minus (–) preceding the dot indicates a negative rho.

Table 4/III. WISC Verbal IQ vs 8 s of EEG power (autospectra) for 3 conditions: Resting I, mental Arithmetic and Resting II for all subjects (n = 83), significant rhos

		Frequency bands															
		3	5	7	9	11	13	15	17	19	21	23	25	27	29	31	33
Resting I																	
Prefrontal	left																
	right							•									
Lat. frontal	left									•		•					
	right																
Frontal	left										•	•	•				
	right																
Central	left						•										
	right																
Temporal	left																
	right																
Post-temporal	left																
	right																
Parietal	left																
	right																
Occipital	left																
	right																
Mental Arithmetic																	
Prefrontal	left											•					
	right											•			•		
Lat. frontal	left						●					●					
	right							•				•			–•		
Frontal	left											●					
	right							•				●					
Central	left				•	•	●										
	right					•						•		•			
Temporal	left						●										
	right					•											
Post-temporal	left																
	right																
Parietal	left					•											
	right					•											
Occipital	left																
	right																
Resting II																	
Prefrontal	left																
	right						•										
Lat. frontal	left						●					•					
	right																
Frontal	left		●				•										
	right		●	•		•	●	•	•	•	●	●					
Central	left	●	•				●	•									
	right	•	•			•	●					•					
Temporal	left	●				•	●										
	right		•			•	●										
Post-temporal	left						•										
	right	●	●	•			●										
Parietal	left	●	●				●	●						•			
	right	●	●				■	•									
Occipital	left						•										
	right	●	●				•										

• Rho with p < 0.05 (0.22–0.27); ● rho with p < 0.01 (0.28–0.35); ● rho with p < 0.001 (0.36–0.42); ■ rho with p < 0.0001 (> 0.42).
A minus (–) preceding the dot indicates a negative rho.

Table 4/IV. WISC Performance IQ vs 8 s of EEG power (autospectra) for 3 conditions: Resting I, mental Arithmetic and Resting II for all subjects (n = 83), significant rhos

		Frequency bands															
		3	5	7	9	11	13	15	17	19	21	23	25	27	29	31	33
Resting I																	
Prefrontal	left						•										
	right																
Lat. frontal	left						•										
	right																
Frontal	left																
	right																•
Central	left						●										
	right																
Temporal	left																
	right																
Post-temporal	left																
	right																
Parietal	left						•										
	right						•										
Occipital	left						●					•	•	•		•	
	right						●					•					
Mental Arithmetic																	
Prefrontal	left																
	right																
Lat. frontal	left																
	right																
Frontal	left	−•															
	right	−•				•											
Central	left						•	●				•					
	right						●	•									
Temporal	left						•										
	right						•										
Post-temporal	left																
	right																
Parietal	left											●					
	right					•						•					
Occipital	left						●				•	●	•				
	right											•					
Resting II																	
Prefrontal	left													−•			
	right																
Lat. frontal	left																
	right											−•					
Frontal	left						•										
	right																
Central	left						●										
	right						●										
Temporal	left						●										−•
	right																
Post-temporal	left																
	right																
Parietal	left						●										
	right						•										
Occipital	left						●						•				
	right	•					●		•								

• Rho with p < 0.05 (0.22–0.27); ● rho with p < 0.01 (0.28–0.35); ● rho with p < 0.001 (0.36–0.42); ■ rho with p < 0.0001 (> 0.42).
A minus (−) preceding the dot indicates a negative rho.

Tables 4/III–4/V show the pattern obtained for the correlations between the same set of EEG scores and the 3 WISC IQ scores: Verbal IQ, Performance IQ and Full-Scale IQ. Of these, table 4/III, for Verbal IQ, shows the smallest degree of similarity of patterns of significant relationships among the 3 conditions, Resting I showing the weakest relationships. Resting I, in fact, shows the weakest relationships throughout, and the problem surrounding the variability of the mental state of the subject during a resting condition is well known.

Table 4/IV shows the relationship between Performance IQ and the 13-Hz activity, with particular emphasis in the occipital areas, while Full-Scale IQ (table 4/V) shows primarily 13-Hz activity correlations.

This first analysis showed primarily that the study indeed had validity but needed further refining. It indicated, first of all, that 8 s of EEG under different conditions showed a considerable amount of reliability which, however, could improve. Particular frequency bands have emerged as furnishing the strongest relationships, among which are the dominant alpha band (the 11-Hz band); the 13-Hz band, a frequency with heretofore unknown relationships; the 23-Hz band which also had no previously known correlations; and the 29-Hz band containing a large number of negative relationships with intellectual scores. Furthermore, inspection of the patterns of significance obtained for all the 8 conditions revealed that the largest number of correlations occurred in the mental Arithmetic condition.

A second set of analyses was performed using 8 s of EEG data obtained during only the mental Arithmetic condition for the purpose of comparing autospectral and cross-spectral values (fig. 4/1–4/5). Autospectral values are represented by dots and cross-spectral values by lines in these figures. Only auto- and cross-spectral values significant beyond the 0.05 levels are shown.

Figures 4/1a and 4/2, relating to the 11-Hz band, show interesting bilateral relationships primarily concerning the verbal subtests and, among the performance subtests, Picture Completion and Block Design.

Figures 4/1b and 4/3 show the relationships of the data pertaining to the 13-Hz activity. The significant pattern is not as generalized. More involved are the left temporal and lateral frontal areas of the verbal subtests. They show some strong central parietal relationships on the left side for Block Design and Object Assembly.

The 23-Hz activity shown in figures 4/1c and 4/4 again shows more relationship with the verbal subtests in the central anterior areas and with the performance subtests in the parietal areas. For this frequency there is a

Table 4/V. WISC Full-Scale vs 8 s of EEG power (autospectra) for 3 conditions: Resting I, mental Arithmetic and Resting II for all subjects (n = 83), significant rhos

		Frequency bands															
		3	5	7	9	11	13	15	17	19	21	23	25	27	29	31	33
Resting I																	
Prefrontal	left						•										
	right																
Lat. frontal	left						•	•		●	•	•					
	right					•											
Frontal	left						•	•			•						
	right																
Central	left						●										
	right																
Temporal	left						•			•							
	right																
Post-temporal	left																
	right																
Parietal	left						•										
	right						•										
Occipital	left						•										
	right						•					•					
Mental Arithmetic																	
Prefrontal	left															•	
	right																
Lat. frontal	left						●					•					
	right					•		•							−•		
Frontal	left					•						•					
	right					●	•	•				•					
Central	left					●	●					•					
	right					●	●					•		•			
Temporal	left					•	●										
	right					•											
Post-temporal	left						•										
	right					•											
Parietal	left					•	•					●					
	right					●	•					•					
Occipital	left					•	•										
	right											•					
Resting II																	
Prefrontal	left																
	right																
Lat. frontal	left						●										
	right					•											
Frontal	left		•			•	●								−•		
	right					●	●				•						
Central	left	•	•			•	■	•									
	right	•	•			•	●	•			•						
Temporal	left	•				•	●										
	right						●										
Post-temporal	left						●										
	right	•	•				●										
Parietal	left	•	●				■	●				•					
	right	•	●				■										
Occipital	left		•			•	●					•					
	right	●	●				●										

• Rho with p < 0.05 (0.22–0.27); ● rho with p < 0.01 (0.28–0.35); ● rho with p < 0.001 (0.36–0.42); ■ rho with p < 0.0001 (> 0.42).
A minus (−) preceding the dot indicates a negative rho.

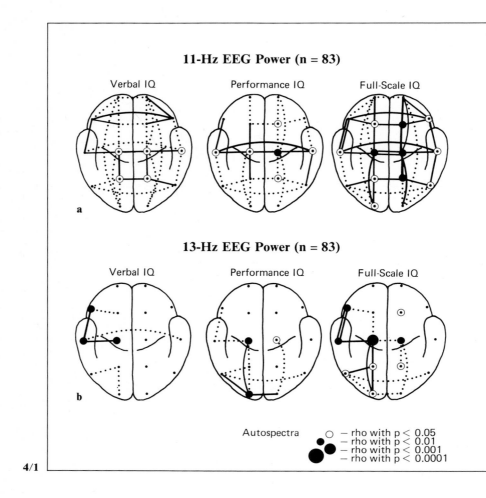

11-Hz EEG Power (n = 83)

Verbal IQ   Performance IQ   Full-Scale IQ

a

13-Hz EEG Power (n = 83)

Verbal IQ   Performance IQ   Full-Scale IQ

b

Autospectra   ○ — rho with p < 0.05
               — rho with p < 0.01
               — rho with p < 0.001
               — rho with p < 0.0001

greater proportion of relationships in the right side in contrast to the previous frequencies.

For the 29-Hz activity, figures 4/1d and 4/5 show the significant negative relationships which do not have a clear consistent pattern except for a number of negative relationships present in the Information and Similarities subtests and reflected in Verbal IQ and then again in Full-Scale IQ, the main contributors being the 2 above-mentioned subtests.

This second set of analyses confirms the greater dimensionality offered by the spectral analysis method with clusters of significant relationships organized in specific patterns related to cognitive variables.

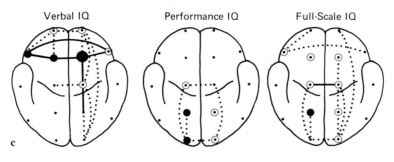

23-Hz EEG Power (n = 83)

Verbal IQ   Performance IQ   Full-Scale IQ

c

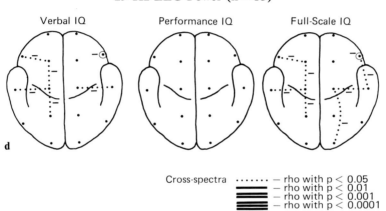

29-Hz EEG Power (n = 83)

Verbal IQ   Performance IQ   Full-Scale IQ

d

Cross-spectra ······· — rho with p < 0.05
━━━━━ — rho with p < 0.01
━━━━━ — rho with p < 0.001
▬▬▬▬ — rho with p < 0.0001

Fig. 4/1a–d. WISC IQ scores vs 11-, 13-, 23- and 29-Hz EEG power (both auto- and cross-spectra) of 8-second EEG obtained while performing mental Arithmetic for all subjects used (n = 83), significant rhos.

Fig. 4/2. WISC subtests' scores vs 11-Hz EEG power (both auto- and cross-spectra) of 8-second EEG obtained while performing mental Arithmetic for all subjects used (n = 83), significant rhos.

Fig. 4/3. WISC subtests' scores vs 13-Hz EEG power (both auto- and cross-spectra) of 8-second EEG obtained while performing mental Arithmetic for all subjects used (n = 83), significant rhos.

Fig. 4/4. WISC subtests' scores vs 23-Hz EEG power (both auto- and cross-spectra) of 8-second EEG obtained while performing mental Arithmetic for all subjects used (n = 83), significant rhos.

Fig. 4/5. WISC subtests' scores vs 29-Hz EEG power (both auto- and cross-spectra) of 8-second EEG obtained while performing mental Arithmetic for all subjects used (n = 83), significant rhos.

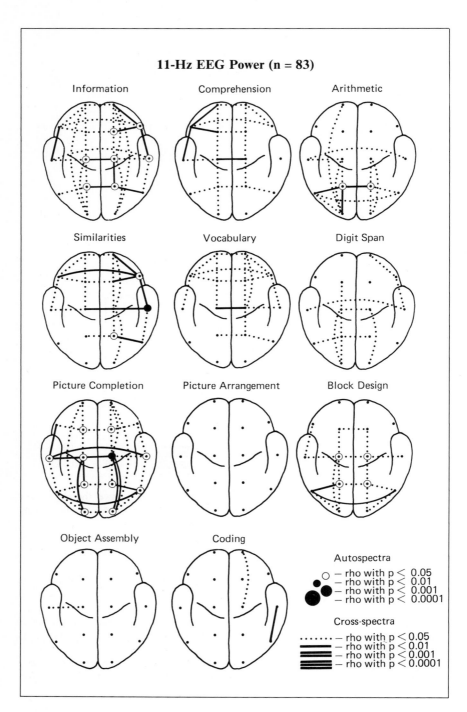

Fig. 4/2. Legend page 55.

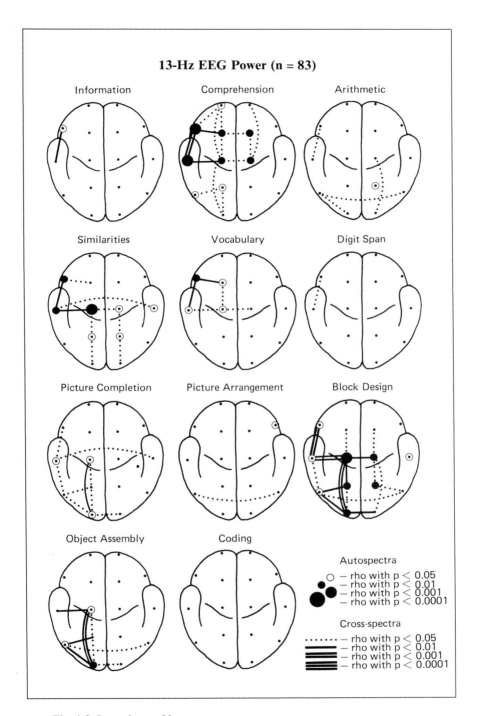

Fig. 4/3. Legend page 55.

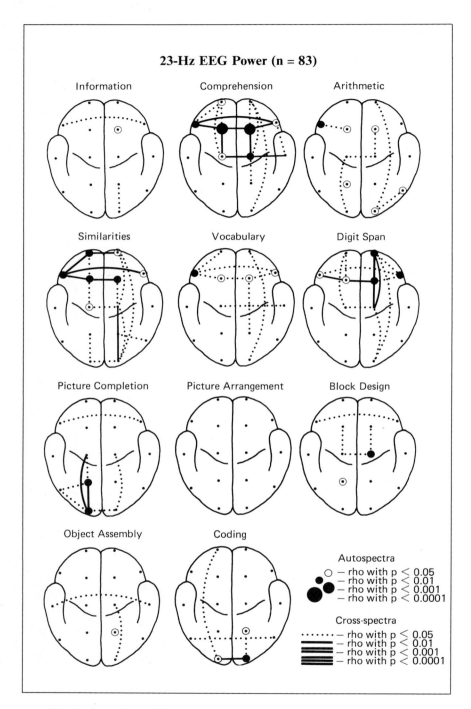

Fig. 4/4. Legend page 55.

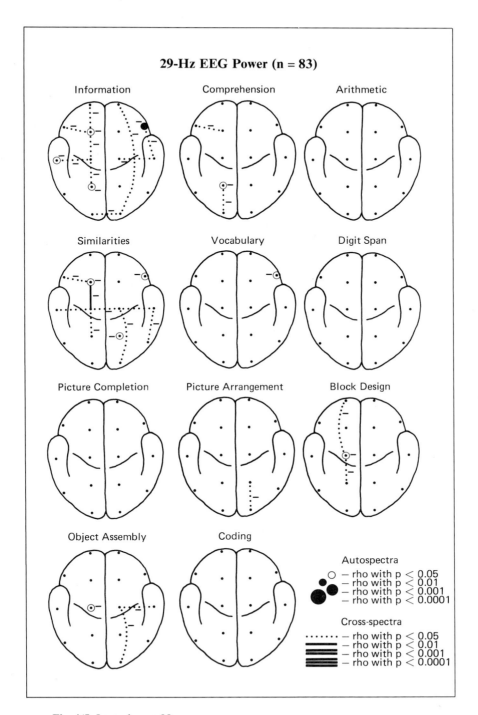

Fig. 4/5. Legend page 55.

Table 4/VI. Intercorrelation among and between WISC subtests and IQ scores in the original standardization sample for 13.5-year-old subjects. Reproduced by permission from the Manual for the Wechsler Intelligence Scale for Children, copyright by the Psychological Corporation [*Wechsler*, 1949]

	Information	Comprehension	Arithmetic	Similarities	Vocabulary	Digit Span	Picture Completion	Picture Arrangement	Block Design	Object Assembly	Coding B	Mazes	Verbal Score
Comprehension	0.61												
Arithmetic	0.59	0.46											
Similarities	0.67	0.61	0.50										
Vocabulary	0.74	0.60	0.46	0.66									
Digit Span	0.39	0.28	0.40	0.34	0.38								
Picture Completion	0.35	0.25	0.26	0.36	0.31	0.23							
Picture Arrangement	0.35	0.31	0.25	0.44	0.41	0.18	0.35						
Block Design	0.48	0.33	0.35	0.45	0.42	0.29	0.51	0.42					
Object Assembly	0.29	0.13	0.20	0.31	0.33	0.13	0.55	0.42	0.63				
Coding B	0.38	0.32	0.34	0.33	0.37	0.24	0.23	0.35	0.35	0.38			
Mazes	0.39	0.21	0.36	0.35	0.32	0.25	0.26	0.29	0.28	0.33	0.27		
Verbal Score[1]	0.80	0.68	0.59	0.74	0.75	0.44	0.38	0.43	0.50	0.31	0.42	0.40	
Performance Score[2]	0.51	0.37	0.38	0.52	0.51	0.29	0.55	0.51	0.65	0.68	0.42	0.39	0.56
Full-Scale Score[3]	0.73	0.58	0.55	0.71	0.70	0.42	0.51	0.53	0.64	0.52	0.48	0.44	–

[1] Digit Span omitted; [2] Mazes omitted; [3] Digit Span and Mazes omitted.

Prior to this research, there have been efforts to understand brain functions through attempts to localize intellectual components (e.g. Wechsler subtests) by studying the relationship of impairment in the performance of these subtests occurring in conjunction with localized brain lesions. Since this area of investigation dealt with higher cortical functions, animal studies were not feasible and experimental lesions in humans were not possible.

The field was therefore relegated to clinical studies of existing brain damage or surgical interventions with insurmountable experimental problems such as: (1) difficulty in verifying the extent of the lesion until after autopsy; (2) lack of control of the extent of the lesion with a consequent difficulty in grouping the subjects for analysis; (3) in the case of surgical ablations, investigation was dependent upon an 'unhealthy' brain with possible anomalous changes such as compensatory migration of functions.

Among the investigations dealing with the Wechsler tests, *Reitan* [1955] and later *Kløve* [1959] studied the feasibility of determining the lateralization of brain damage on the basis of differentials in deficits between verbal and performance subtests. Except for minor differences in the data obtained for individual subtests, data from the two studies showed consistent differentials. The fact that for most subtests significant deficits occurred in patients with both left and right hemispheric damage remained unexplained and was regarded implicitly or explicitly as of secondary importance to the main effect of being able to differentiate lateralization of damage.

These studies stem from a long line of thought [*Giannitrapani*, 1967] localizing language functions in the left hemisphere. This investigator demonstrated a historical difficulty in the scientific acceptance of contralaterality consequent to the existence of the corticospinal decussation in the pyramid. Once Broca's findings became available, this contralaterality became embodied in the concept of whole hemispheric dominance without heed being paid to the warnings dating as far back as 1871 when *Jackson* [1958] postulated that when speaking of hemispheric dominance one should always specify the function which was being referred to as being dominant.

In analyzing both *Reitan's* [1955] and *Kløve's* [1959] graphs one can determine that Object Assembly, for instance, which of all Wechsler subtests shows for the WISC the highest correlation with Performance IQ (table 4/VI), does not show the highest loss consequent to right hemispheric damage. Conversely, Digit Span, which among the verbal subtests shows the lowest correlation with the verbal scale (table 4/VI), shows the greatest loss consequent to left hemispheric damage. The only possible general conclusion short of arguing sampling problems, reliability of the criterion of localization methods, peripheral deficits affecting performance or age differences in the sample, arguments which are all partially true, is that functions are not entirely unilaterally arranged as generally expressed or implied. The present data shows a complex pattern of lateralization which supports this latter notion.

Alternately, *McFie* [1960], in his series of patients with localized cerebral lesions, found a different pattern of impairment for the Wechsler subtests. The localization of this impairment shows, for instance [*McFie*, 1969], a deficit in the performance of the digit symbol (Coding) subtest in all analyzed brain regions (right and left frontal, temporal and parietal). This is perhaps because of a generalized reduction in the speed of motor performance in this timed test.

From these findings it would be erroneous to conclude that the localization of the digit symbol task is to be found in the entire brain on the basis of this 'achievement' measure without any electrophysiological understanding of the processes involved in the task. It is for this reason that one should refrain from drawing brain diagrams (with sulci and gyri) identifying brain areas with Wechsler subtest labels as if these labels had any electrophysiological reality.

Without being able to yet understand the electrophysiological processes involved, the present data are descriptive of functionally related electrophysiological activity and, as such, open a new area of investigation permitting a closer scrutiny of the process.

The distribution of significant correlations obtained can be compared to the intercorrelation matrix developed by *Wechsler* [1949] for his standardization sample of 13.5-year-olds, reproduced here for ease of comparison (table 4/VI). *Wechsler's* intercorrelation matrix shows correlations of 0.60 or higher for all comparisons involving Information, Comprehension, Similarities and Vocabulary. Inferences from table 4/VI could not go beyond accepting the face validity of such intercorrelations. Figure 4/2 reveals electrophysiological similarities of 11-Hz activity of these 4 subtests involving central and anterior areas. Figure 4/3, for 13-Hz activity, reveals another component involving temporal and lateral frontal derivations while figure 4/4, for 23-Hz activity, recapitulates some of the patterns of significance of the 11-Hz activity. The 23-Hz band could be including the second harmonic of the activity shown in the 11-Hz band, but it shows unique features of diversity in degrees of significance. Lateralization is also an issue, e.g. Similarities showing higher intercorrelations on the left side for 23 Hz and on the right side for 11 Hz while the opposite is true for Picture Completion.

Without making an attempt to analyze all relationships for which current neuropsychological knowledge furnishes support, it can be noted that the lower level of relationship among the verbal subtests for Arithmetic and Digit Span (table 4/VI) is also observable in figures 4/2, 4/3 and 4/4.

Among the performance subtests, Block Design correlates highest with Verbal IQ, and the portion of the electrophysiological activity which could be responsible for this similarity is also observable in these figures while the performance component of Block Design can be inferred as resulting from a parieto-occipital activity as shown again by these figures.

Prior to obtaining the data, it was theorized that this type of analysis of intellectual functions might be more sensitive to performance components of mental abilities. The data instead show greater sensitivity to verbal components and furthermore a virtual absence of significant activity for Picture Arrangement. On the other hand, the intercorrelation of 0.63 between Block Design and Object Assembly (table 4/VI) seems to be expressed in figure 4/3 by the left central occipital relationship of the 13-Hz activity.

These preliminary sets of analyses produced findings that, even though in need of refinement, offered enough support of existing neuropsychological knowledge to warrant closer and more extensive scrutiny.

References

Giannitrapani, D.: Developing concepts of lateralization of cerebral functions. Cortex *3:* 353–370 (1967).

Giannitrapani, D.; Roccaforte, P.: Reliability measurements of EEG components in different behavioral states; in Matejcek, Schenk, Quantitative analysis of the EEG. Proc. 2nd Symp. Study Group for EEG Methodology, Jongny-sur-Vevey 1975, pp. 761–772.

Jackson, J.H.: Selected writings of Hughlings Jackson (Basic Books, New York 1958).

Kløve, H.: Relationship of differential electroencephalographic patterns to distribution of Wechsler-Bellevue scores. Neurology, Minneap. *9:* 871–876 (1959).

McFie, J.: Psychological testing in clinical neurology. J. nerv. ment. Dis. *131:* 383–393 (1960).

McFie, J.: The diagnostic significance of disorders of higher nervous activity; in Vinken, Bruyn, Handbook of clinical neurology, vol. 4, pp. 1–12 (Am. Elsevier, New York 1969).

Reitan, R.M.: Certain differential effects of left and right cerebral lesions in human adults. J. comp. physiol. Psychol. *48:* 474–477 (1955).

Wechsler, D.: WISC manual, Wechsler Intelligence Scale for Children (Psychological Corp., New York 1949).

5 Auto- and Cross-Spectra of the Right-Preferent Sample

'... the measurement is not completed until its result enters our consciousness ... the last step is, at the present state of our knowledge, shrouded in mystery ...'
E.P. Wigner on scientific measurement

One of the main questions that arose at this time was the lateralization of functions. Most of the findings in both the first set of analyses (tables 4/I–4/V) and the second set of analyses (fig. 4/1–4/5) indicated, except for the 23-Hz activity, a stronger relationship on the left side. Since this sample was composed of a group which included left-preferent, mixed and right-preferent subjects, it was felt desirable to separate the data into different groups in order to see whether this homologous asymmetry in the data would be maximized. The next analyses then were restricted to the 56 subjects who constituted the right sample of the subject pool.

For these analyses a set of data was studied, comparable to the data analyzed in chapter 4, i.e. 8 s of EEG obtained during 3 conditions: Resting I, mental Arithmetic and Resting II. For the cross-spectral data, analysis was restricted to the mental Arithmetic condition as in chapter 4. The only difference then between the 2 chapters is that chapter 4 deals with a subject sample (n = 83), containing both left- and right-handed subjects, while chapter 5 (n = 56) is constituted of right-preferent subjects only.

Tables 5/I–5/III show Wechsler Intelligence Scale for Children (WISC) IQ scores obtained for the right-handed sample for the autospectral values. Again we see a basic pattern of consistencies for the 3 IQ scores, a degree of consistency which is not entirely satisfactory, especially in Performance IQ (table 5/II) where the differences between the first and second Resting conditions are too great to consider an 8-second sample acceptable. There is a negative cluster of significant relationships in the second Resting condition which remains unexplained at this time. In the Full-Scale IQ, however, a much higher degree of significance was obtained, the largest dot (■) representing significance at the 0.0001 level. It should be noted that the rho

Table 5/I. WISC Verbal IQ vs 8 s of EEG power (autospectra) for 3 conditions: Resting I, mental Arithmetic and Resting II for the right-preferent subjects (n = 56), significant rhos

		\multicolumn{16}{c}{Frequency bands}

		3	5	7	9	11	13	15	17	19	21	23	25	27	29	31	33
\multicolumn{18}{c}{**Resting I**}
Prefrontal	left									•		●	•				
	right											•					
Lat. frontal	left					•	•			•		•	•				
	right						●	•		•	•						
Frontal	left						•				•	•	•				
	right											•	•				
Central	left					•	●										
	right				•	•	•					•	•				
Temporal	left					•	●										
	right					•	●										
Post-temporal	left																
	right																
Parietal	left																
	right																
Occipital	left																
	right																
\multicolumn{18}{c}{**Mental Arithmetic**}
Prefrontal	left											•	•				
	right											●	•	•			
Lat. frontal	left			•		•	•	●				•					
	right						•		•		•	•					
Frontal	left					•	•	●					•	•			
	right					•	•	•				•					
Central	left					●	●	●				•					
	right					•	•	•						•		•	
Temporal	left					●	•	●									
	right			•	•	●	•	●									
Post-temporal	left					•	•										
	right					•											
Parietal	left					●	•										
	right					•											
Occipital	left																
	right																
\multicolumn{18}{c}{**Resting II**}
Prefrontal	left						●										
	right					•	●										
Lat. frontal	left					•	•										
	right					●	•									−•	
Frontal	left		●			•	●	•	•		•					−•	
	right		●	•		●	■		•		●	●					−•
Central	left	●	●			•	●	•									
	right	•	●			•	■				●						
Temporal	left				•	•	●									−•	
	right		•			•	●									−•	−•
Post-temporal	left					•	•										
	right	●	●	•			•									−•	−•
Parietal	left	•	■			•	●	●									
	right	•	●	•		•	●	●									
Occipital	left		•														
	right	•	•														−•

• Rho with p < 0.05 (0.26–0.34); ● rho with p < 0.01 (0.35–0.42); ● rho with p < 0.001 (0.43–0.47); ■ rho with p < 0.0001 (> 0.48).
A minus (–) preceding the dot indicates a negative rho.

Table 5/II. WISC Performance IQ vs 8 s of EEG power (autospectra) for 3 conditions: Resting I, mental Arithmetic and Resting II for the right-preferent subjects (n = 56), significant rhos

		Frequency bands															
		3	5	7	9	11	13	15	17	19	21	23	25	27	29	31	33
Resting I																	
Prefrontal	left						•			•						•	
	right				•											•	
Lat. frontal	left						•								•		
	right				•												•
Frontal	left						•				•						
	right																
Central	left						•					•	•	•			
	right																
Temporal	left						•										
	right																
Post-temporal	left																
	right																
Parietal	left											•					
	right																
Occipital	left						•		•	•	•	●	●			●	
	right																
Mental Arithmetic																	
Prefrontal	left																
	right																
Lat. frontal	left																
	right					•											
Frontal	left	−•				•											
	right					•	•										
Central	left					●	●					•	•				
	right					●	●					•	•				
Temporal	left					•											
	right					•	•										
Post-temporal	left																
	right		−•			•											
Parietal	left					•	•					●	•				
	right					●	•					●					
Occipital	left					•	•					●	•	•			
	right					•						●					
Resting II																	
Prefrontal	left																
	right																
Lat. frontal	left									−•		−•	−●	−•		−•	−•
	right											−●	−●	−●			−•
Frontal	left					•	•										
	right					•											−•
Central	left					•	●										
	right					•	●										−•
Temporal	left									−•		−●	−●	−●	−●	−●	−●
	right											−•	−•			−•	−●
Post-temporal	left													−•			−•
	right																
Parietal	left																−•
	right																−•
Occipital	left						•					•					
	right	•							•			•					

• Rho with p < 0.05 (0.26–0.34); ● rho with p < 0.01 (0.35–0.42); ● rho with p < 0.001 (0.43–0.47); ■ rho with p < 0.0001 (> 0.48).
A minus (−) preceding the dot indicates a negative rho.

Table 5/III. WISC Full-Scale IQ vs 8 s of EEG power (autospectra) for 3 conditions: Resting I, mental Arithmetic and Resting II for the right-preferent subjects (n = 56), significant rhos

		Frequency bands															
		3	5	7	9	11	13	15	17	19	21	23	25	27	29	31	33
Resting I																	
Prefrontal	left						●			●		●	•			•	
	right																
Lat. frontal	left					•	●			●	•	•	•	•			
	right					•	●	•			•	•					
Frontal	left					•	●	•		•	●	•	•				
	right						•					•					
Central	left					•	●				•						
	right					•	●	•				•	•				
Temporal	left					•	●										
	right					•	●	•									
Post-temporal	left																
	right																
Parietal	left											•					
	right						•					•					
Occipital	left												•				
	right												•				
Mental Arithmetic																	
Prefrontal	left													•			
	right																
Lat. frontal	left					•	●					•					
	right					●		•									
Frontal	left					•	●					•					
	right					●	●	•									
Central	left				•	■	■		•		•	•					
	right				•	●	■	•				●					
Temporal	left				•	●	■										
	right				•	●	●										
Post-temporal	left					•	•										
	right					•											
Parietal	left					●	•	•				•					
	right					●	•	•				•					
Occipital	left					•	•										
	right					•											
Resting II																	
Prefrontal	left						•										
	right						•										
Lat. frontal	left					•	•						−•	−•	−•	−•	
	right					•							−•	−•	−•	−•	−•
Frontal	left		•			●	●	•							−●		−•
	right		•			●	●	•			•				−•		−●
Central	left	•	•			●	■	●							−•		−•
	right	•	●			●	■	●			•				−•		−•
Temporal	left					●	●						−•	−•	−●	−●	−●
	right					•	●								−•	−•	−●
Post-temporal	left						•								−•		−•
	right	●	●				•								−•		−●
Parietal	left		●			•	●	●									−•
	right		●			•	■	•			•				−•		−•
Occipital	left		●			•	•										
	right	●	●												-		−●

• Rho with p < 0.05 (0.26–0.34); ● rho with p < 0.01 (0.35–0.42); ● rho with p < 0.001 (0.43–0.47); ■ rho with p < 0.0001 (> 0.48). A minus (–) preceding the dot indicates a negative rho.

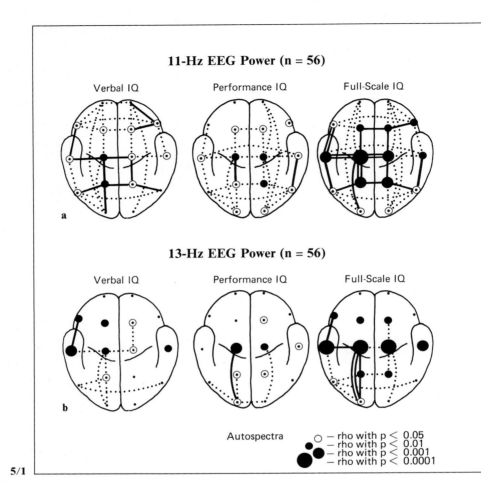

11-Hz EEG Power (n = 56)

Verbal IQ   Performance IQ   Full-Scale IQ

a

13-Hz EEG Power (n = 56)

Verbal IQ   Performance IQ   Full-Scale IQ

b

Autospectra
- ○ — rho with $p < 0.05$
- ● — rho with $p < 0.01$
- ● — rho with $p < 0.001$
- ● — rho with $p < 0.0001$

5/1

values necessary to reach significance are larger in this third set of analyses where the sample was reduced (cf. table 6/I). The dots, therefore, indicate a level of significance (not a rho value) equal to that of the first set of analyses (tables 4/I–4/V).

Continuing the exploration of the feasibility of utilizing this sample of right-handed subjects, figures 5/1–5/5 show the pattern obtained for this sample for both autospectra and cross-spectra of the mental Arithmetic condition in the 4 selected frequency bands: 11, 13, 23 and 29 Hz. Comparison of figure 5/1a with figure 4/1a for the 11-Hz activity shows relatively little change except for an increase of significance in the Full-Scale IQ

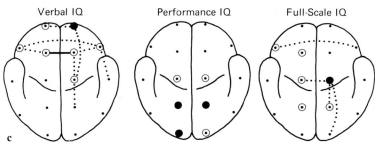

23-Hz EEG Power (n = 56)

Verbal IQ   Performance IQ   Full-Scale IQ

c

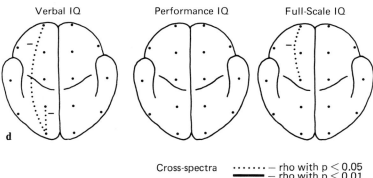

29-Hz EEG Power (n = 56)

Verbal IQ   Performance IQ   Full-Scale IQ

d

Cross-spectra ······ — rho with p < 0.05
— rho with p < 0.01
— rho with p < 0.001
— rho with p < 0.0001

Fig. 5/1a-d. WISC IQ scores vs 11-, 13-, 23- and 29-Hz EEG power (both auto- and cross-spectra) of 8-second EEG obtained while performing mental Arithmetic for the right-preferent subjects (n = 56), significant rhos.

Fig. 5/2. WISC subtest scores vs 11-Hz EEG power (both auto- and cross-spectra) of 8-second EEG obtained while performing mental Arithmetic for the right-preferent subjects (n = 56), significant rhos.

Fig. 5/3. WISC subtest scores vs 13-Hz EEG power (both auto- and cross-spectra) of 8-second EEG obtained while performing mental Arithmetic for the right-preferent subjects (n = 56), significant rhos.

Fig. 5/4. WISC subtest scores vs 23-Hz EEG power (both auto- and cross-spectra) of 8-second EEG obtained while performing mental Arithmetic for the right-preferent subjects (n = 56), significant rhos.

Fig. 5/5. WISC subtest scores vs 29-Hz EEG power (both auto- and cross-spectra) of 8-second EEG obtained while performing mental Arithmetic for the right-preferent subjects (n = 56), significant rhos.

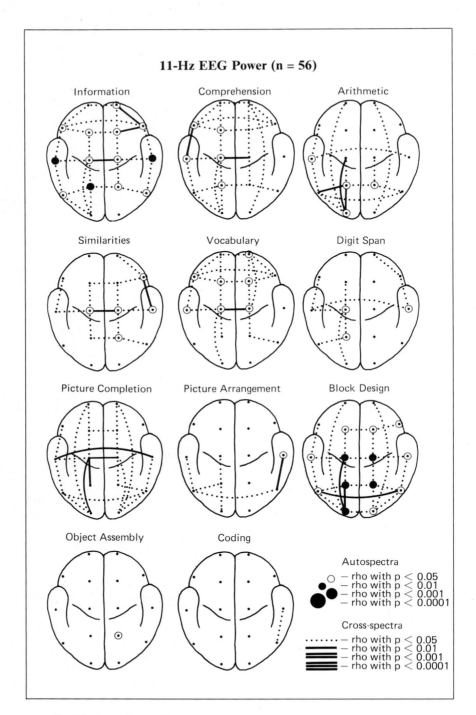

Fig. 5/2. Legend page 69.

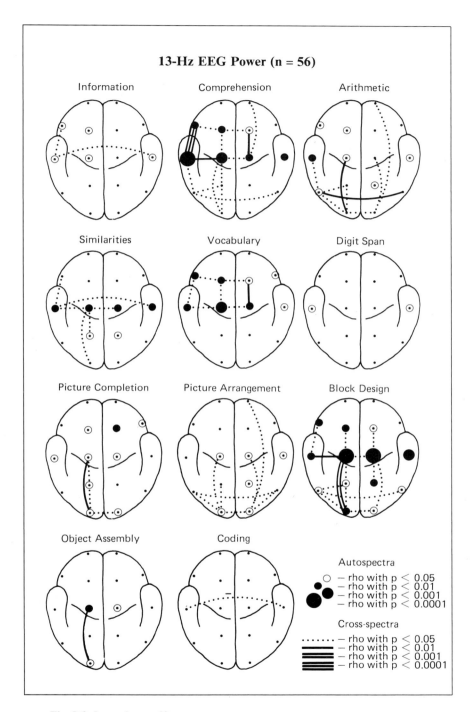

Fig. 5/3. Legend page 69.

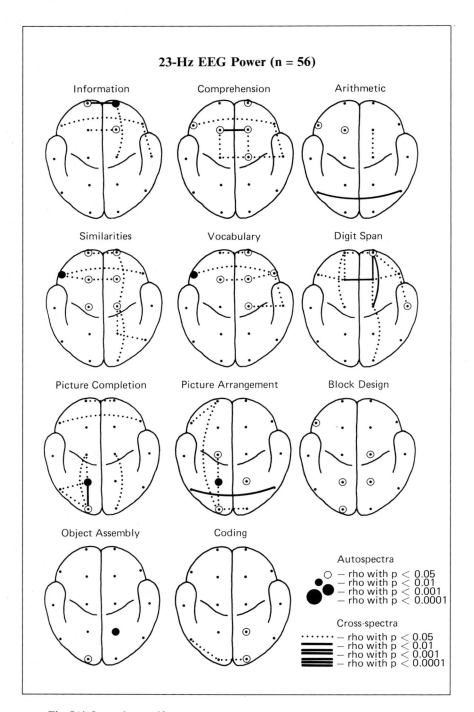

Fig. 5/4. Legend page 69.

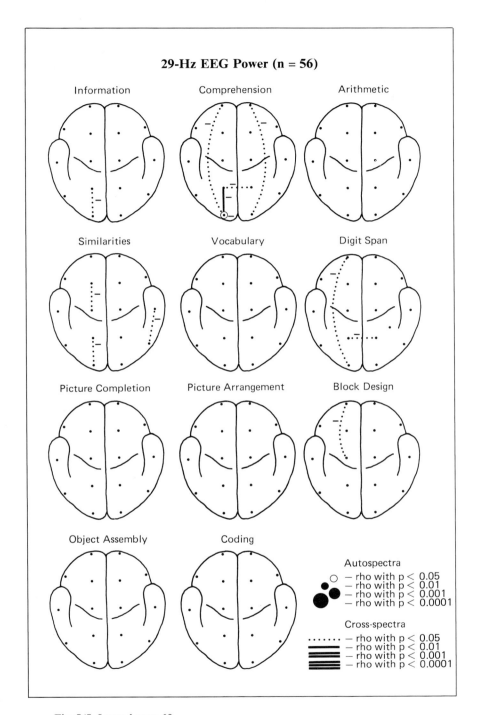

Fig. 5/5. Legend page 69.

correlations. Comparison of figure 5/2 with 4/2, again with 11-Hz activity for the subtests, indicates perhaps a decrease in significance in some of the subtests and reveals no new pattern.

The same accrues for the comparison of figure 5/1b with figure 4/1b, while in the comparison between figure 5/3 and 4/3 there seems to be considerable increase in significance in the 13-Hz relationship in this newly analyzed sample (fig. 5/3). Of interest, not having been observed in figure 4/3, is a cascade of activity in Picture Arrangement, apparently originating in the 2 occipital areas and relating to the activity of more anterior regions.

Extrapolating about the different roles that 11- and 13-Hz activity have in the processing of higher intellectual functions, the 11-Hz activity seems to relate to a broader network of relationships in the brain. The 13-Hz activity seems to concentrate on the execution of specific functions, for instance, the left temporal and lateral frontal in Comprehension (fig. 5/1b); the central to occipital relationship in Digit Span in the same figure; and the cascade in Picture Arrangement, also in the same figure. While in figure 5/2 for the 11-Hz the relationships are weaker, they are greater in number and perhaps involve memory functions, as for instance, expressed in Digit Span involving the temporal, lateral frontal and prefrontal derivations.

The 23-Hz activity is shown in figures 5/1c and 5/4. The 23-Hz activity was chosen because of its number of correlations in a frequency range in which otherwise there was a low concentration of correlations with intellectual variables. A comparison of figure 5/1c with figure 4/1c shows a decrease in relationships with equal levels of significance, and this pattern was shown also in a comparison between figure 5/4 and 4/4. It was at first believed that 23-Hz activity could have been a harmonic of the 11-Hz activity, but it was found here that the distribution of 23 Hz is quite different, and the lateralization is also different, the 23-Hz being primarily lateralized to the right side while the 11-Hz was lateralized to the left side. The reason for this is not understood at this time, but it points to the dimensionality of the technique, and it cautions the reader against facile interpretation of the function of a given area based on a single measure such as an evoked potential or a measure of blood flow which would be representative of gross changes in the metabolic activity of a brain area and not be sensitive to differentials which are observed here between different EEG frequency bands.

The 29-Hz activity is shown in figures 5/1d and 5/5. It was included here, as mentioned before, because of an early interest in 29-Hz activity which seemed to correlate with pathology [*Giannitrapani and Kayton,* 1974] and was later found to correlate negatively with intellectual functions as shown in table 7/II. The significant relationships are weak, and the pattern shown in the larger sample of n = 83 (fig. 4/1d) is not upheld in figure 5/1d where the sample was reduced. Further inspection of figure 5/1d also shows a low level of concordance between that figure and 4/5, pointing to the low value of these correlations. The significant fact remains, however, that the correlations are all negative, and one can conclude that the 29-Hz activity has physiological significance which is opposite to the significance of the other frequencies studied.

The investigator at this point was in a very interesting position, being on one hand overwhelmed by the richness of the material and on the other hand somewhat concerned about the degree of reliability of 8-second periods. The first consideration permitted beginning to look at psychological parameters which were emerging as relating to physiological parameters and stimulating some of the thinking that was later developed and expanded by *Liberson* in chapter 13. The other consideration, however, led to the conclusion that further analysis should have as a basic measure much more reliable data, and to that effect, all subsequent work relied upon a multiple of 8 s obtained by averaging the 8 conditions tested and thus obtaining one score for these eight 8-second periods constituted by 64 s of EEG. Thus, the following chapters will deal with this averaged data.

Reference

Giannitrapani, D.; Kayton, L.: Schizophrenia and EEG spectral analysis. Electroenceph. clin. Neurophysiol. *36:* 377–386 (1974).

6 Left-Preferent Sample

'As many men, so many minds; every one his own way.'
Terence (185–159 BC)

It became obvious from inspection of the data in chapter 4 that the correlations between EEG spectra and mental functions in a sample having both left- and right-preferent subjects, even though by and large symmetrical, tended to be greater on the left side. This asymmetry could be related to brain dominance, and an attempt was made to clarify this issue in chapter 5 by selecting a right-handed sample. The results were inconclusive, the data still showing a tendency for the correlations to be higher on the left side, but a significant increase in this asymmetry which could have been predicted consequent to the elimination of the left preferent subjects in the sample did not occur. The final test of the brain dominance hypothesis required selecting a left-preferent sample, computing correlations for that group and determining whether for this group correlations were higher on the right side.

In order to pursue this issue, 20 left-preferent subjects having a laterality preference score in the left-preferent third of the range were selected. Sample correlations were performed between Wechsler Intelligence Scale for Children (WISC) Full-Scale IQ scores and the EEG scores for the Voice, Arithmetic and patterned Vision conditions as well as for the average of all 8 conditions. The 13-Hz activity was selected for these comparisons since it was shown to be the frequency with the highest correlations.

The Spearman rhos computed are shown in table 6/I. The rhos for the mental Arithmetic condition are directly comparable to the 13-Hz rhos of mental Arithmetic in table 4/V for the full subject sample and table 5/III for the right preferent sample. The rhos obtained for the average of the 8 conditions can be compared to the full-scale autospectra rhos in figure 4/1b for the full subject sample and figure 5/1b for the right-preferent sample. Further comparisons can be made in the appropriate cells of table 7/I for the Voice, Arithmetic and patterned Vision conditions and in the rhos obtained for the 13-Hz activity in table 9/XIV for the average of the 8 conditions.

Table 6/I. Left-preferent sample (n = 20). Selected rhos between WISC Full-Scale IQ and 13-Hz EEG power (8-second duration) for the Voice, Arithmetic and patterned Vision conditions and for the mean of the 8 conditions. Significance levels of n = 20 apply. For comparison with the significance levels in tables 5/III, 7/I and 9/XIV and figure 5/1b of the right-preferent data (n = 56) and table 4/V and figure 4/1b of the full sample data (n = 83), significance levels are given for the 3 sample sizes:

	n = 20	n = 56	n = 83
$p < 0.05$	0.38	0.26	0.22
$p < 0.01$	0.53	0.35	0.28

		Conditions			
		Voice	Arithmetic	patterned Vision	mean of 8 conditions
Lat. Frontal	left	0.12	0.33	0.15	0.33
	right	−0.10	0.13	0.16	0.18
Frontal	left	−0.02	−0.12	−0.12	−0.02
	right	−0.01	−0.08	−0.07	−0.08
Central	left	0.22	0.19	0.24	0.25
	right	0.23	−0.05	−0.10	0.10
Temporal	left	−0.02	0.34	0.13	0.01
	right	−0.26	−0.16	0.06	−0.11

Comparisons are somewhat hampered by the fact that the 3 sets of tables (n = 83, n = 56, n = 20) require progressively larger rho values for a given level of significance. For this reason the 3 separate sets of values required are included for comparison in table 6/I.

Comparisons show no support for the hypothesis that the asymmetries of rhos obtained, showing a larger proportion of higher rhos on the left side, is due to brain dominance as measured by the laterality preference tests used in this study. Since this hypothesis has such a clear lack of support, no further correlations were computed for the left preferent group.

Two main possibilities may account for this seeming lack of distribution of asymmetrical scores in the left-preferent sample. One is that this asymmetry of distribution of intelligence related rhos is indeed unrelated to brain dominance or that either the measurement or definition (or both) of brain dominance are in need of substantive revision.

The finding that data from a left-preferent group is not distributed in mirror image fashion when compared to a right-preferent group is not new, but it is always surprising, so strong are the expectations for such contralaterality to occur. In the present investigator's research, spectral distribution of EEG activity differences between left and right preferents is overwhelmingly not mirror image [*Giannitrapani,* 1979]. A review of the findings dealing with aphasia can be found in *Hécaen* [1962].

Notable is the work of *Conrad* [1949] who found that most of the aphasic left-handed patients had damage in the left hemisphere. He concluded that left-handedness implied a less developed lateralization rather than a mirror image of right-handedness. The data of the present study did not directly test this hypothesis since the correlations depend on group data. Of the three laterality preference groups of the present study the data of the mixed-preferent group had the largest sigma, perhaps in support of *Critchley's* [1953] analysis postulating the existence of five different mechanisms for achieving a condition of non-right preference.

Giannitrapani [1975] invoked *Yakovlev's* notion of torque in interpreting alleged migration of functions in the left preferents, not to homologous areas but to areas adjacent to homologous areas. *Yakovlev* [1972] explained that the cerebral hemispheres do not originate from a bilateral structure and assume only secondarily the positional symmetry of two hemispheres. The early neural tube is primarily ablateral, and the cerebral cortex retains a statistical 'torque' in a numerical distribution of efferent cortical fibers from both hemispheres to the right side of the neuraxis. This is evidenced by a consistent priority of the left pyramidal tracts to cross 90% of the time at higher level and in larger number of fibers to the right side of the spinal cord [*Yakovlev and Rakić,* 1966].

The variance between individuals, however, even in the differential between crossed fibers on the left and right sides of the brain in the same individual, is so great as to render untenable the 90% crossed fiber assumption when studying a clinical case. It is possible that through the noninvasive technique of EEG spectral analysis, studied under the appropriate conditions, information could be obtained in vivo for this and other postulated fiber decussations in man such as those of the auditory system.

It is hypothesized here that vestiges of the above-mentioned torque are to be found also in the cortex and may be responsible for that portion of individual asymmetry of cerebral function which is of genetic origin.

Accepting as given the right motoric preference and the left cerebral preference for speech in the human species, the brains of the subjects having anomalies to this architectonic distribution of functions would contain an inherent greater plasticity because of the developmentally more recent occurrence of such anomaly. In this situation, when such an individual is presented with a task which is presented to all members of the species, such an individual has a greater opportunity to solve the problem in a novel way and at the same time is penalized by not having as readily available to him the circuitry which the species has available for the performance of that task. It is perhaps for this reason that, while 5% of the population is left-preferent, using the same criterion for laterality measurement, more than 5% of mentally retarded, epileptics, mentally ill, athletes, musicians, artists, dancers, MENSA members and Nobel prize winners are left preferents.

Each member of the human species when presented with a new task, be it responding to sounds or understanding speech, has to find a way for his/her brain to process such information. For the new organism this is a novel situation which can be solved only if the cytoarchitecture for the solution of these tasks is available. The availability of this cytoarchitecture furnishes only the possibility for solving the task but does not solve the task per se. The burden of the solution is on the individual, and the probability and the stereotypy of the solution is greater if the circuitry for the solution of this task was available to phylogenetically older species. This fact is well demonstrated at the cortical level, e.g. in the highly predictable localization of motor functions in the precentral gyrus and of the visual projection areas in the occipital lobes. The difficulty, therefore, in localizing higher cortical functions is perhaps due to the higher degree of plasticity of those portions of the neocortex which preside over the more complex functions in man.

The interest in the issue of brain dominance in all its ramifications is exemplified by the proliferation of literature in this field to such an extent that an exhaustive survey of the literature is practically impossible. The genesis of the current thinking in this field was described by *Giannitrapani* [1967]. Because of this interest and because of the above-mentioned plasticity and consequent poor understanding of distribution of functions, inferences have been drawn from insufficient data. As an example, there is no support in this study for *Kimura's* [1973] assertion that melodies are processed predominantly by the right temporal lobe (fig. 15/3). Her conclusions were drawn from the slight left-ear advantage (with alleged primarily crossed fibers) found when 2 different melody segments were simultaneously presented to the 2 ears. The asymmetry she noted might be due not to the mechanism governing perception of melody in this artificial experimental situation but possibly to a dominant role that the right temporal lobe has in the search for structure as shown in chapter 16. This interpretation might complement *Darwin's* [1974] criticisms of the conclusions usually drawn from dichotic listening studies.

In conclusion, the concept of hemispheric dominance is entirely too broad to be of any value, and the choice of a rationale concerning the higher correlations between EEG activity and mental functions on the left side of the brain should be deferred until the mechanism governing this activity is better understood. The possible rationales range from the most peripheral to the most central. To mention but one such rationale, the reader should be reminded of the greater reliability observed in the activity in most areas of the left side of the brain (fig. 3/4), a fact which alone could be responsible for the higher correlations obtained on the left side in this study. This explanation, however, does not further the understanding of the asymmetrical reliability invoked above which remains to be studied. This asymmetry in reliability could be either the cause or the effect of dominant utilization of brain structures, and if it were the former this mechanism could help in understanding the physiological mechanism of the genesis of dominance.

References

Conrad, K.: Über aphasische Sprachstörungen bei hirnverletzten Linkshändern. Nervenarzt *20:* 148–154 (1949).

Critchley, M.: The parietal lobes, p. 397 (Hafner, New York 1953).

Darwin, C.J.: Ear differences and hemispheric specialization; in Schmitt, Worden, The neurosciences: Third Study Program, pp. 57–64 (MIT Press, Cambridge 1974).

Giannitrapani, D.: Developing concepts of lateralization of cerebral functions. Cortex *3:* 353–370 (1967).

Giannitrapani, D.: The notion of torque in the distribution of cerebral functions; in Symp. Philosophical Questions about the Physical Notion of Force (Int. School of Philosophy of Science, Erice 1975).

Giannitrapani, D.: Laterality preference, electrophysiology and the brain. Electromyogr. clin. Neurophysiol. *19:* 105–123 (1979).

Hécaen, H.: Clinical symptomatology in right and left hemispheric lesions; in Mountcastle, Interhemispheric relations and cerebral dominance, pp. 215–243 (Johns Hopkins Press, Baltimore 1962).

Kimura, D.: The asymmetry of the human brain. Sci. Am. *228:* 70–78 (1973).

Yakovlev, P.: A proposed definition of the limbic system; in Hockman, Limbic system mechanisms and autonomic function, pp. 241–283 (Thomas, Springfield 1972).

Yakovlev, P.; Rakić, P.: Patterns of decussation of bulbar pyramids and distribution of pyramidal tracts on two sides of the spinal cord. Trans. Am. Neur. Ass., pp. 366–367 (1966).

III Correlation Matrices of the Right-Preferent Data

'... we have to develop a dualist-interactionist philosophy according to which the self-conscious mind has an identity and activity that are not entirely dependent on brain events, these events being under a determining and controlling influence from the self-conscious mind.'
Sir *John Eccles*

7 Right-Preferent Data

'Some people say that the heart is the organ with which we think and that
it feels pain and anxiety. But it is not so. Men ought to know that from the
brain and from the brain only arise our pleasures, joys, laughters, and tears.
Through it, in particular, we think, see, hear, and distinguish the ugly from
the beautiful, the bad from the good, the pleasant from the unpleasant ...
To consciousness the brain is messenger.'
Hippocrates (460?–?377 BC)

Chapters 7–11 discuss the matrices of correlations between EEG power
scores (autospectra) and intellectual variables for the right-preferent sample
which was introduced in chapter 5 with both auto- and cross-spectral data.
Chapter 12 reviews an additional set of matrices which were obtained by
correlating the same EEG power scores with intellectual factor scores rather
than with intellectual subtest scores. This further refinement permits a better understanding of the role the different brain areas have in the exercise of
different functions.

By studying EEG spectra under different conditions of stimulation or
different intellectual states, it is possible to make inferences about the
changes in the functional role of brain areas dependent upon the location of
the changes in electrical activity. Within that experimental paradigm, however, it is not possible to differentiate between the changes that are central
or peripheral to the task in question. In the case, for instance, of a comparison between a neutral condition and an intellectual task requiring verbal
output, changes may be due to any number of factors, some of them conceptual, some of them related to visualization of the task, and many of them
related to different aspects of verbal performance (e.g. lexical, phonemic,
motoric).

On the other hand, by studying a single set of EEG spectra obtained
under a given condition and by correlating it with different intellectual
parameters, the different patterns of correlations obtained constitute a more

direct measure of the brain activity which is either necessary, a facilitator or a sine qua non of the intellectual parameter in question. By inspecting the patterns of these coefficients, one can then draw conclusions about which brain activity (which brain area, which frequency band) is positively or negatively related to which intellectual function. This latter strategy is utilized here.

The initial sample was comprised of 83 subjects of whom a relatively large number were left- and mixed-preferent. In subsequent analyses the right-preferent subjects were selected from the original sample. The bulk of the analyses were performed on the right-preferent sample.

To better evaluate the contribution of each condition to the overall correlation values, table 7/I presents in a condensed form the significant rhos obtained for the EEG of the 8 conditions separately when compared with the scores of the Wechsler Intelligence Scale for Children (WISC) Full-Scale IQ. Shown in each cell are 8 of these rhos, 1 for each of the 8 conditions, arranged as explained in the footnote. Please note that the data in this table pertaining to the Resting I, mental Arithmetic and Resting II conditions are shown in table 5/III, and that a portion of the data pertaining to the mental Arithmetic condition is included in the Full-Scale IQ diagrams of figure 5/1.

One can see at a glance the high degree of comparability of the different conditions which justified using the average EEG for the 8 conditions as a representative score. In particular, attention of the reader is directed to the 13-Hz activity of the central areas which indicates that each of the 8 conditions studied shows a consistently high relationship with WISC Full-Scale IQ scores. This finding is in support of the existence of EEG frequency components which occur in the brain under a variety of conditions and which, if not *responsible* for intellectual functions, are indicative of the *possibility* for executing intellectual functions.

The EEG power scores used in chapters 8–13 were obtained by summing one 8-second period for each of the 8 conditions for a total of 64 s of EEG. The same EEG scores were used in all the matrices to correlate them with the different intellectual scores in order to determine which portion of the EEG activity and which brain area is related to a given intellectual measure.

Please note that, while the spectral data available consisted of 17 frequency bands from 0 to 34 Hz, the correlational analyses of chapters 4 and 5 and table 7/I include 16 frequency bands from 2 to 34 Hz because of limitations in the computational matrices. The 1-Hz band (0–2 Hz) had

Table 7/I. WISC Full-Scale IQ vs 8 s of EEG power (autospectra), n = 56. Significant rhos for each of the 8 conditions (8 s each) are represented in each cell. Values for each condition are positioned as explained below in the arrangement scheme

Frequency bands

Brain areas		3	5	7	9	11	13	15	17	19	21	23	25	27	29	31	33
Prefrontal	left						2 2 1					2 1	1			1 1	
	right						1			2				1				
Lat. frontal	left					1 1 1 1	2 1 3 3	2		2	1	1	1	1-1	-1	-1	-1
	right			1	1	1 1	1 2 1 2	1			1	1	-1	-1	-1	-1	-1
	right				2	1 2	2 1	1 1		1 1 1		1	-1	-1			
Frontal	left	1	1			1 1 1 2 1 1 2	3 2 2 1 3 2 1 2	1 1 1 1 2 1	1	1 1 1	2	1	1		-2		-1
	right	1 1	1		1	2 1 2	1 2 2 3 3 2 3 2	1 1 2 1	2	1	1	1	1		-1		-2
Lat. frontal	left	1	1	1	1	1 2 1 1 2 2 1 4	3 3 3 3 4 3 3 4	1 1 2 2 1	-1		1	1	1		-1		-1
	right	1	2		1	1 2 1 1 3 2 1 3	2 3 3 3 4 3 3 4	1 1 1 2 1	1		2	1			-1		-1
Temporal	left					1 1 1 1 2 1 3 3	3 1 3 3 3 2 2 4	2					-1	-1	-3	-2	-2
	right					1 1 1 1 1 2 1 2	2 1 3 3 2 2 1 3	1 1 1		1		2			-1	-1	-2
Post-temporal	left					1 1	2	1	1						-1		-1
	right	2	2			1 1	1 1 1 1 1 2	1	1				1		-1		-2 -1
Parietal	left	1 1	2			1 1 3	1 2 2 3 2 1 2	1 2 1 2 1	1			1 1					-1 -1
	right	1 1	2	1		1 1 2 1 1 1 1 3	1 1 1 3 4 2 1 2	1 1 1 1			1	1 1		-1	-1		-1 -1
Occipital	left	1	2			1 1 1 1	1 1 1 1 1 1	1	1			1	2 1 1 1 1			1	-1
	right	1 1	2	1		1 1 -1	1					1	1				-2

1 = Rho with p < 0.05; 2 = rho with p < 0.01; 3 = rho with p < 0.001; 4 = rho with p < 0.0001.

Arrangement scheme: Resting I   Noise   Music   Voice
                     Resting II Diffuse Visual Arithmetic

been discarded on the incorrect assumption that slow frequencies would not be related to mental activity, and the 33-Hz band (32–34 Hz) was included to explore new territory. Those analyses demonstrated that the 33-Hz band contributed little information, and exploratory research revealed that the 1-Hz band yielded significant data. Subsequent correlational analyses dealing with 64 s of EEG were designed, therefore, to include frequencies from 0 to 32 Hz in 16 frequency bands.

It is important to reemphasize that throughout the book, unless otherwise specified, the matrices of rhos compared within a chapter are obtained from identical sets of EEG scores. The differences in the correlation coefficients of different matrices, therefore, are due to the differences in rank of the scores obtained by the subjects in the performance of an intellectual task. The term rank is used here because the correlation coefficients used were rhos which are rank order correlation coefficients. This correlation formula makes no assumption of equal intervals within either EEG spectral values or WISC subtest scores.

There are 19 correlation matrices based on the averages of the 8 EEG conditions. The first shows the relationships between EEG and age (chapter 8). The next 14 show the relationships between EEG and each of the WISC weighted subtest scores as well as the 3 IQ scores (chapter 9 with the exclusion of table 9/XV). The last 4 show the relationships between EEG and each of the 4 tests developed in our laboratory (chapter 10). Additional discussion of the same significant rhos but organized according to the brain areas in which they are found is presented in chapter 11. Chapter 12 utilizes the same set of EEG scores and presents additional matrices obtained by correlating these EEG scores with WISC factor scores rather than WISC subtest scores.

For clarity, the matrices show only the rhos that are significant beyond the 0.05 level of confidence. Because of the number of correlations computed and the consequent presence of significant rhos obtained purely by chance, only clusters of correlations are discussed and not isolated rhos.

In addition to the matrices of EEG scores representing the average of the 8 conditions, matrices representing the EEG obtained from each 8-second condition separately will be discussed in each section whenever pertinent. These latter matrices for the separate conditions, however, are not shown in tabular form except for those shown in chapters 4 and 5 and tables 7/I and 9/XV.

8 EEG Frequency Changes with Age

'... Nature has contrived the brain as a counterpoise to the region of the heart with its contained heat and has given it to animals to moderate the latter compounding it of earth and water ... the brain then tempers the heat and seething of the heart.'
Aristotle from *Parts of Animals* (384–322 BC)

The ontogenetic development of the normal EEG was studied with precomputer technology by *Lindsley* [1938]. A brief summary of his age findings which would relate to the sample of the present study follows: (1) a gradual increase in the frequency of dominant activity from birth to puberty, and (2) a gradual decrease in EEG amplitude during the same period. While there was no expectation of finding significant changes in the narrow yet developmentally diverse age range of this study (a 3-year span), the correlations between EEG power and age in months were computed to determine some EEG baselines against which to compare the correlations with intellectual scores. Even though Wechsler Intelligence Scale for Children (WISC) weighted scores were used (normalized for age), the confounding of 2 variables, i.e. a growing electrophysiological organism and the increase in intellectual performance with age, could still be present.

Giannitrapani [1975] demonstrated that in the narrow age range from 11 to 13 years the correlations between EEG power and age were overwhelmingly negative, indicating a decrease in power with increase in age. The correlations were significantly negative in 2 broad bands, from 1 to 8 Hz and from 20 to 28 Hz. Table 8/I shows the significant rhos obtained. It is quite evident from this table that all significant correlations are negative. A decrease of delta and theta with age was already known [later observed by *John* et al., 1980; *Gasser* et al., 1983a] while the decrease of high beta activity had not been previously described. All of these decreases have later been observed in the same age group by *Pratusevich* et al. [1981]. The alpha band in table 8/I does not show any significant correlations with the age group of the sample. There are some indications [*Katada* et al., 1981] that the alpha reaches a developmentally mature level at about age 10. The absence of positive correlations for the dominant alpha band (11-Hz band for this group) would confirm no further increase in this activity in the 11- to 13-year-old range while the absence of negative correlations would indicate that the decline of alpha activity, which occurs with age in a portion of the population, has not yet begun. It is possible, of course, that for certain individuals in this sample the alpha activity is still maturing while for others it is already decreasing, but in general the statement can be made that in 11- to 13-year-olds dominant alpha activity is at a plateau.

In the full matrix of 256 correlations only 17 are positive and, of these, 12 (none of them reaching the 0.05 level of significance) occur in the 29-Hz band. The characteristics of the 29-Hz activity are unique in many respects and will be discussed wherever applicable (cf. table 8/II).

Subdivision of this matrix into the separate conditions' matrices, 1 for each EEG condition of 8 s duration (not shown), yields basically the same information with the following exceptions:

(1) 8 significant negative correlations in the 11-Hz band in the mental Arithmetic condition, indicating that the residual dominant alpha component present during the performance of mental Arithmetic decreases with age in this 11- to 13-year-old sample.

Table 8/I. Age in months (11–0 through 13–11) vs 64 s of EEG power (autospectra) for the right-preferent sample (n = 56), significant rhos all of which are negative as indicated

		Frequency bands															
		1	3	5	7	9	11	13	15	17	19	21	23	25	27	29	31
Prefrontal	left	−•											−•	−•			
	right			−•									−•	−●	−●		
Lat. frontal	left	−•	−•	−●	−•							−•	−●	−●	−•		
	right			−•										−•			
Frontal	left		−•	−●	−•								−●	−●	−•		
	right	−•	−●	−●	−•									−•	−•		
Central	left			−●	−●	−•											
	right	−•	−●	−•	−•												
Temporal	left	−•	−●	−●										−•			
	right		−•	−•	−•					−•			−•	−•	−•		
Post-temporal	left	−●	−•	−●						−•			−•	−•	−●		−•
	right	−●	−●	−•									−•	−•	−•		
Parietal	left	−●	−●	−●	−•												
	right	−●	−●	−•													
Occipital	left	−●	−•														
	right	−•															

• Rho with p < 0.05 (0.26–0.34); ● rho with p < 0.01 (0.35–0.42); ● rho with p < 0.001 (0.43–0.48); ■ rho with p < 0.0001 (> 0.48). A minus (–) preceding the dot indicates a negative rho.

(2) The 29-Hz activity shows, among all brain areas and conditions, only 1 significant negative correlation (rho = −0.31 for the Music condition in the right prefrontal area) and 3 of the 4 positive significant correlations found among all the matrices obtained for age. 2 of the 3 significant positive coefficients occurred in the 2 central areas during the mental Arithmetic condition (rho = +0.30 and +0.27), and most of the remaining conditions show their highest positive correlations in these brain areas as well. The pattern of the coefficients obtained for the 29-Hz band indicates that this is the only frequency which is positively related with age within the ages studied.

The fact that the bulk of EEG power in this sample is negatively correlated with age is relevant not only as a confirmation of early observations. It acquires special meaning when attempting to separate the role of maturation from mental abilities. These two dimensions in their various manifestations are usually positively related. Finding EEG power negatively related

Table 8/II. Distribution of negative rhos in 16 frequency bands (16 brain areas pooled) regardless of significance. Note the overwhelming incidence of negative rhos for age and the relatively greater incidence of negative rhos in the non-WISC tests because of their not having been age-standardized. Note also the overall inverse relationship in the incidence of negative rhos between 29-Hz activity and the other frequencies

	Distribution of negative rhos															
	1	3	5	7	9	11	13	15	17	19	21	23	25	27	29	31
Age	16	16	16	16	16	16	13	15	16	16	16	16	16	16	4	15
Spatial Relations	1	6	4	11	9	5	1	4	4	7	11	2	4	7	16	10
Symbol Manipulation	1	10	11	16	7					2	2	5	7	11	14	11
Verbal Analogies	5	10	9	14	1			3	4	4	5	5	10	14	8	15
Psychomotor Efficiency	14	16	16	16	15	6	1	13	6	7	6	12	12	14	1	14
WISC subtests																
Information		1	1	6			1	2		5	2	4	8	10	14	11
Comprehension		1					2	2	2	4	1		5	9	16	9
Arithmetic		2	2	9	4										1	1
Similarities		1	1	8	5		2	2	4	2	1		5	9	14	10
Vocabulary				1			2	2	4	2	1	6	8		15	11
Digit Span	1	3	4	9			1			3	1	1	2	1	14	6
Picture Completion		2	3	10	4	3		5	2	3		1	2	2	3	2
Picture Arrangement	5	9	14	16	6	3	2	1		1	2	6	10	5	10	1
Block Design		3	2	1	1			2	2	4	3			2	12	11
Object Assembly	2	4	13	16	15			7	8	9	9	8	9	11	16	8
Coding	14	14	14	9			8	12	12	4	1	6	6	9	3	6
Verbal IQ		1		4				2		2	1		5	7	14	7
Performance IQ	2	10	10	12	2		2	5	3	7	3	5	5	8	12	6
Full-Scale IQ	1	4	3	8	2			1		3	2		2	7	15	7

with age and positively related with mental functions (as shown later) presents an unprecedented and welcome possibility to differentiate the role of the 2 parameters.

To elucidate further the age-mental function differential present in the incidence of negative rhos, table 8/II shows the distribution of negative rhos present in each frequency band for each matrix studied for the subject sample (n = 56). Note that the maximum value obtainable in each cell is 16, i.e. the 16 brain areas in which a negative rho could occur for that particular frequency band.

The lack of positive relationship between age and weighted WISC scores speaks well for the pragmatic age normalization performed by Wechsler to obtain the weighted scores. This finding affirms that the positive relationship between EEG power and intellectual scores is not a reflection of maturational processes as is the case in the data of *Gasser* et al. [1983b], but a resultant of processes which could be regarded as intellectual-specific. The search for the specific intellectual correlate to the broad finding of an EEG-intellectual activity relationship continues.

The fact that the age factor had an opposite role from the intellectual factors raises the possibility of the existence of even higher relationships between EEG power and intellectual factors, had a narrower age group been selected.

References

Gasser, T.; Möcks, J.; Lenard, H.G.; Bächer, P.; Verleger, R.: The EEG of mildly retarded children: developmental, classificatory and topographic aspects. Electroenceph. clin. Neurophysiol. *55:* 131–144 (1983a).

Gasser, T.; Lucadou-Müller, I. von; Verleger, R.; Bächer, P.: Correlating EEG and IQ: a new look at an old problem using computerized EEG parameters. Electroenceph. clin. Neurophysiol. *55:* 493–504 (1983b).

Giannitrapani, D.: Spectral analysis of the EEG; in Dolce, Künkel, CEAN, computerized EEG analysis, pp. 384–402 (Fischer, Stuttgart 1975).

John, E.R.; Ahn, H.; Prichep, L.; Trepetin, M.; Brown, D.; Kaye, H.: Developmental equations for the electroencephalogram. Science *210:* 1255–1258 (1980).

Katada, A.; Ozaki, H.; Suzuki, H.; Suhara, K.: Developmental characteristics of normal and mentally retarded children's EEG. Electroenceph. clin. Neurophysiol. *52:* 192–201 (1981).

Lindsley, D.B.: Electrical potentials of the brain in children and adults. J. gen. Psychol. *19:* 285–306 (1938).

Pratusevich, Y.M.; Solov'ev, A.V.; Kvasov, G.I.: Utilization of factor analysis for the evaluation of ontogenetic and functional changes in the electrical activity of the brain. J. Hyg. Epid. Microbiol. Immunol. *25:* 259–269 (1981).

9 WISC Matrices

'Appearances to the mind are of four kinds.
Things either are what they appear to be;
or they neither are, nor appear to be;
or they are, and do not appear to be;
or they are not, and yet appear to be.
Rightly to aim in all these cases is the wise man's task.'
Epictetus (circa AD 60)

The intercorrelation matrices between the EEG spectral scores (64-second average of 8 conditions) and the 11 Wechsler Intelligence Scale for Children (WISC) subtests as well as the 3 major IQ scores are analyzed in this chapter. Each intellectual variable tested will be discussed with an interpretation of the significant rhos present in the matrices of correlations between EEG and intellectual variables.

As mentioned in chapter 3, separate matrices of intercorrelations were obtained for each subtest score for each of the 8 conditions in which the EEG was obtained and for the 64-second average of the 8 conditions. For the sake of brevity, only the matrices for the 64-second averages are shown in total while the salient features of the matrices for the 8 separate conditions are discussed in the text with only the mental Arithmetic matrix shown in tabular form. A portion of this information was discussed in *Giannitrapani* [1981].

Information

This subtest contains questions formulated to tap the subject's range of information. With Vocabulary, it is the most 'achievement' among achievement tests because it measures previously aquired knowledge. The major objection to its use is that an individual's fund of knowledge is measurably related to education and cultural opportunities. *Wechsler* [1949] included it in the battery because of its high correlation with total score. This subtest can be interpreted as indicating the alertness of the person toward the world around him, and among all subtests it correlates highest with Verbal and Full-Scale IQ.

Table 9/I shows a number of significant positive correlations between EEG spectra and the Information subtest scaled scores. There is an unexpected cluster of positive correlations in the lowest frequencies (1–5 Hz band) in central and parietal areas with higher correlations on the right side. This cluster is unexpected because the presence of low frequency activity in the EEG is traditionally regarded as occurring with poor cortical functioning, pathology or sleep. The type of clustering would indicate that this is not a random phenomenon. It is observed to a greater or lesser extent in all subtests (except Arithmetic) of the Verbal Scale as well as Picture Completion and Block Design. This 1-Hz activity seems to be a necessary correlate of capacity for verbal activity.

The next cluster of significant correlations is in 3 bands, 9–13 Hz, stronger in the 11-Hz. All significant activity up to and including 11 Hz shows a clear lateralization, higher positive coefficients being shown on the right side from frontal to parietal areas. The 11-Hz activity is in the same band (10–12 Hz) and perhaps of identical frequency as dominant alpha activity.

A third cluster of significant correlations in the prefrontal areas is at 23 Hz and higher. These correlations with a high beta activity will be found also in the Similarities and Picture Completion subtests. They may serve a role in the frontal lobes' scanning for hypotheses. In contrast with lower frequency activity, the beta coefficients obtained for the prefrontal activity are higher on the left side.

An interesting cluster of negative correlations occurs in the high beta frequencies in the other brain areas, rarely reaches significance but appears often in relation to other subtests especially in the 29-Hz frequency band. The negativity of the high beta frequencies will be discussed later under comprehension.

Inspection of matrices of the individual EEG conditions (not shown) reveals similar patterns throughout with one notable exception. The 29-Hz band for the Noise condition shows a solid column of negative coefficients (except for the prefrontal areas) and weak positive correlations in the lower significant bands shown above. The Noise condition also shows the greatest number of other significant negative coefficients in the high beta frequencies when compared with the matrices of the other conditions for this subtest.

Comprehension

The Comprehension subtest requires practical information and an ability to evaluate appropriate responses to situations. *Wechsler* avoided specifying what functions might be involved in the performance of this task. It seems that one of the unique features of Comprehension is not only the ability to elicit responses from within but more important the ability to evaluate the appropriateness of each elicited response, i.e. to form a judgment regarding which response is appropriate or relevant within the given context and at what point to terminate the search for a response. It could be called a test of contextual appropriateness. It does not correlate as high with Verbal IQ as do the Similarities and Vocabulary subtests.

The Comprehension subtest, table 9/II, among all the WISC subtests or even among the other intellectual scores used in the study, correlates most highly, by far, with the EEG scores used. There is a broad band of significant correlations from 1 to 23 Hz with the exclusion of the 19-Hz band. There is great similarity with the pattern obtained for the Information subtest except that for Comprehension the correlations are higher in the 13-Hz band and on the left side. It is as if the reasoning required for efficient performance in the Comprehension subtest is utilizing the presence of EEG frequencies in a broad spectrum and in all brain areas with the notable exception of the occipital areas. Correlations in the 13-Hz band go beyond the 0.001 level of significance, the highest ones being in the left and right central areas with a rho = 0.49 and 0.48, respectively.

The 2 negative correlations in the 31-Hz band in right posterior areas belong to the cluster of negative correlations in the high frequencies, which for the most part remain below significance levels. Inspection of the matrices of the individual conditions (not shown) reveals a similarity in the patterns with the following notable exceptions:

(1) The patterned Vision condition shows a cluster of negative coefficients in the occipital areas for the 27- to 33-Hz bands [a decrease in all frequencies in the occipital areas for the patterned Vision condition has already been demonstrated by *Giannitrapani,* 1970]. This cluster of negative coefficients indicates that persistence or increase of these beta frequencies, when the subject has eyes open and is looking at a geometrical pattern,

Table 9/I. WISC Information vs 64 s of EEG power (autospectra) for the right-preferent sample (n = 56), significant rhos

		Frequency bands															
		1	3	5	7	9	11	13	15	17	19	21	23	25	27	29	31
Prefrontal	left						•						●	•			•
	right						•						•	•	•		•
Lat. frontal	left						●	•									
	right						●	•									
Frontal	left					•	●	•				•	•				
	right	●	•	●		●	•	•					•				
Central	left	•	•				●	•									
	right	●					•	•									
Temporal	left						●									−•	
	right	•	•			●	●	•									
Post-temporal	left																
	right	•	•			•											
Parietal	left	•					•										
	right	•					•	•									
Occipital	left																
	right																

• Rho with p < 0.05 (0.26–0.34); ● rho with p < 0.01 (0.35–0.42); ● rho with p < 0.001 (0.43–0.48); ■ rho with p < 0.0001 (> 0.48).
A minus (–) preceding the dot indicates a negative rho.

Table 9/II. WISC Comprehension vs 64 s of EEG power (autospectra) for the right-preferent sample (n = 56), significant rhos

		Frequency bands															
		1	3	5	7	9	11	13	15	17	19	21	23	25	27	29	31
Prefrontal	left						•	•					•				
	right																
Lat. frontal	left				•		●	●					•				
	right						•	•									
Frontal	left			•	•	●	•	●	•			●	●				
	right		●	●	●	●	•	●	•	•		•	●				
Central	left	●	●			●	●	■	•			•					
	right	•					•	●	•				•				
Temporal	left	•		•	•	•	●	●									
	right	•		•	•	•	•	●									
Post-temporal	left			•		•		•									
	right		•			•											−•
Parietal	left	•	●	•			•	•	•								
	right	•	●	•		•	•										
Occipital	left																
	right																−•

• Rho with p < 0.05 (0.26–0.34); ● rho with p < 0.01 (0.35–0.42); ● rho with p < 0.001 (0.43–0.48); ■ rho with p < 0.0001 (> 0.48).
A minus (–) preceding the dot indicates a negative rho.

Table 9/III. WISC Arithmetic vs 64 s of EEG power (autospectra) for the right-preferent sample (n = 56), significant rhos

		Frequency bands															
		1	3	5	7	9	11	13	15	17	19	21	23	25	27	29	31
Prefrontal	left																
	right																
Lat. frontal	left							●									
	right							•									
Frontal	left							●	•			•	•				
	right							●	•	•							
Central	left							●	•	•							
	right							●	•								
Temporal	left							●	•	•							
	right							●	•								
Post-temporal	left							•		●			•				
	right																
Parietal	left							•		•			•				
	right							•		•							
Occipital	left									•			•	•			
	right									•				•			

• Rho with p < 0.05 (0.26–0.34); ● rho with p < 0.01 (0.35–0.42); ● rho with p < 0.001 (0.43–0.48); ■ rho with p < 0.0001 (> 0.48).
A minus (–) preceding the dot indicates a negative rho.

Table 9/IV. WISC Similarities vs 64 s of EEG power (autospectra) for the right-preferent sample (n = 56), significant rhos

		Frequency bands															
		1	3	5	7	9	11	13	15	17	19	21	23	25	27	29	31
Prefrontal	left												•	•			
	right												•		•		
Lat. frontal	left							•									
	right						•										
Frontal	left						•	•					•				
	right			•			•	•					•				
Central	left	•					•	●									
	right	•					•	●									
Temporal	left						•	•									
	right	•	•				●	●									
Post-temporal	left																
	right	•															
Parietal	left	•															
	right						•	•									
Occipital	left																
	right																

• Rho with p < 0.05 (0.26–0.34); ● rho with p < 0.01 (0.35–0.42); ● rho with p < 0.001 (0.43–0.48); ■ rho with p < 0.0001 (> 0.48).
A minus (–) preceding the dot indicates a negative rho.

Table 9/V. WISC Vocabulary vs 64 s of EEG power (autospectra) for the right-preferent sample (n = 56), significant rhos

		\multicolumn{16}{c}{Frequency bands}
		1	3	5	7	9	11	13	15	17	19	21	23	25	27	29	31
Prefrontal	left						●										
	right						•	•									
Lat. frontal	left					•	●	●									
	right	•				•	●	•									
Frontal	left			•		●	●	●					•	●			
	right	•		●		●	●	●					•	●			
Central	left	•	•			●	●	■									
	right	•				●	●	●						•			
Temporal	left					•	●	•									
	right	●				●	•	●									
Post-temporal	left					•											
	right		•			●	•										
Parietal	left	•	•			•	•	•									
	right	•	•			•	•	•									
Occipital	left																
	right		•														

• Rho with p < 0.05 (0.26–0.34); ● rho with p < 0.01 (0.35–0.42); ● rho with p < 0.001 (0.43–0.48); ■ rho with p < 0.0001 (> 0.48).
A minus (–) preceding the dot indicates a negative rho.

Table 9/VI. WISC Digit Span vs 64 s of EEG power (autospectra) for the right-preferent sample (n = 56), significant rhos

		\multicolumn{16}{c}{Frequency bands}
		1	3	5	7	9	11	13	15	17	19	21	23	25	27	29	31
Prefrontal	left																
	right										•		•		•		
Lat. frontal	left																
	right					•											
Frontal	left						•										
	right						•										
Central	left						•										
	right	•					●										
Temporal	left					•	●										
	right					•	●	●			•		●				
Post-temporal	left																
	right	•	•								•						
Parietal	left	•															
	right	•															
Occipital	left	•															
	right	●	•														

• Rho with p < 0.05 (0.26–0.34); ● rho with p < 0.01 (0.35–0.42); ● rho with p < 0.001 (0.43–0.48); ■ rho with p < 0.0001 (> 0.48).
A minus (–) preceding the dot indicates a negative rho.

Table 9/VII. WISC Picture Completion vs 64 s of EEG power (autospectra) for the right-preferent sample (n = 56), significant rhos

		Frequency bands															
		1	3	5	7	9	11	13	15	17	19	21	23	25	27	29	31
Prefrontal	left										·	·	·	·	●		●
	right	·													·	·	·
Lat. frontal	left	·															
	right																
Frontal	left							·							·		
	right																·
Central	left							●									
	right							·									
Temporal	left	·															
	right	·															
Post-temporal	left																
	right																
Parietal	left							·									
	right							·									
Occipital	left	·						·		·							
	right																

· Rho with p < 0.05 (0.26–0.34); ● rho with p < 0.01 (0.35–0.42); ● rho with p < 0.001 (0.43–0.48); ■ rho with p < 0.0001 (> 0.48). A minus (–) preceding the dot indicates a negative rho.

Table 9/VIII. WISC Picture Arrangement vs 64 s of EEG power (autospectra) for the right-preferent sample (n = 56), significant rhos

		Frequency bands															
		1	3	5	7	9	11	13	15	17	19	21	23	25	27	29	31
Prefrontal	left																
	right																
Lat. frontal	left			–·													
	right			–·	–·												
Frontal	left																
	right									·							
Central	left							·	●	●							·
	right								·	·							
Temporal	left																
	right								·		·						
Post-temporal	left							·									
	right									·							
Parietal	left								·	·							·
	right								·	●	·						
Occipital	left							·		●	·		·	·			
	right									·		·					

· Rho with p < 0.05 (0.26–0.34); ● rho with p < 0.01 (0.35–0.42); ● rho with p < 0.001 (0.43–0.48); ■ rho with p < 0.0001 (> 0.48). A minus (–) preceding the dot indicates a negative rho.

Table 9/IX. WISC Block Design vs 64 s of EEG power (autospectra) for the right-preferent sample (n = 56), significant rhos

		Frequency bands														
		1	3	5	7	9	11	13	15	17	19	21	23	25	27	29	31
Prefrontal	left																
	right																
Lat. frontal	left							●					・				
	right																
Frontal	left			・	・			●	・				・				
	right							・									
Central	left			・			・	●	・								
	right	・	・				・	●	・				・				
Temporal	left							●									
	right							・									
Post-temporal	left			・	・			・		・							
	right							・		・							
Parietal	left	・	・	・			・	・	・	・			・	・			
	right	・	・				・	●									
Occipital	left		・				・	・		・			・	・			
	right																

• Rho with p < 0.05 (0.26–0.34); ● rho with p < 0.01 (0.35–0.42); ● rho with p < 0.001 (0.43–0.48); ■ rho with p < 0.0001 (> 0.48).
A minus (–) preceding the dot indicates a negative rho.

Table 9/X. WISC Object Assembly vs 64 s of EEG power (autospectra) for the right-preferent sample (n = 56), significant rhos

		Frequency bands														
		1	3	5	7	9	11	13	15	17	19	21	23	25	27	29	31
Prefrontal	left																
	right																
Lat. frontal	left																
	right																
Frontal	left																
	right																
Central	left							・									
	right							・									
Temporal	left							・									
	right																
Post-temporal	left																
	right																
Parietal	left																
	right																
Occipital	left													・			
	right																

• Rho with p < 0.05 (0.26–0.34); ● rho with p < 0.01 (0.35–0.42); ● rho with p < 0.001 (0.43–0.48); ■ rho with p < 0.0001 (> 0.48).
A minus (–) preceding the dot indicates a negative rho.

Table 9/XI. WISC Coding vs 64 s of EEG power (autospectra) for the right-preferent sample (n = 56), significant rhos

		Frequency bands														
		1	3	5	7	9	11	13	15	17	19	21	23	25	27	29	31
Prefrontal	left																
	right																
Lat. frontal	left																
	right																
Frontal	left		−•														
	right		−•														
Central	left													•			
	right																
Temporal	left																
	right																
Post-temporal	left																
	right																
Parietal	left																
	right																
Occipital	left				•					•	•		•				
	right										•						

• Rho with p < 0.05 (0.26–0.34); ● rho with p < 0.01 (0.35–0.42); ● rho with p < 0.001 (0.43–0.48); ■ rho with p < 0.0001 (> 0.48).
A minus (–) preceding the dot indicates a negative rho.

Table 9/XII. WISC Verbal IQ vs 64 s of EEG power (autospectra) for the right-preferent sample (n = 56), significant rhos

		Frequency bands														
		1	3	5	7	9	11	13	15	17	19	21	23	25	27	29	31
Prefrontal	left						•	•					•	•			
	right						•	•					•		•		
Lat. frontal	left						●	●					•				
	right						●	•									
Frontal	left			•		•	●	●	•		•	•	●				
	right	•		●		•	●	●	•	•	•	●	•				
Central	left	●	•			•	●	■				•					
	right	●					●	■									
Temporal	left						●	●									
	right	•	•			•	●	■									
Post-temporal	left						•	•									
	right	•	•			•	•										
Parietal	left	•	•				•	•									
	right	•	•				●	●									
Occipital	left																
	right		•														

• Rho with p < 0.05 (0.26–0.34); ● rho with p < 0.01 (0.35–0.42); ● rho with p < 0.001 (0.43–0.48); ■ rho with p < 0.0001 (> 0.48).
A minus (–) preceding the dot indicates a negative rho.

Table 9/XIII. WISC Performance IQ vs 64 s of EEG power (autospectra) for the right-preferent sample (n = 56), significant rhos

		Frequency bands															
		1	3	5	7	9	11	13	15	17	19	21	23	25	27	29	31
Prefrontal	left																
	right																
Lat. frontal	left																
	right																
Frontal	left		−•														
	right																
Central	left							●									
	right							•									
Temporal	left							•									
	right																
Post-temporal	left																
	right																
Parietal	left													•			
	right																
Occipital	left							•		•		•	●	•			
	right												•				

• Rho with p < 0.05 (0.26–0.34); ● rho with p < 0.01 (0.35–0.42); ● rho with p < 0.001 (0.43–0.48); ■ rho with p < 0.0001 (> 0.48). A minus (–) preceding the dot indicates a negative rho.

Table 9/XIV. WISC Full-Scale IQ vs 64 s of EEG power (autospectra) for the right-preferent sample (n = 56), significant rhos

		Frequency bands															
		1	3	5	7	9	11	13	15	17	19	21	23	25	27	29	31
Prefrontal	left												•				
	right																
Lat. frontal	left						•	●									
	right						•	•									
Frontal	left						•	●	•		•	•	•				
	right			•		•	•	■	•	•		•					
Central	left						•	■	•								
	right	•					•	■	•				•				
Temporal	left						•	●									
	right						•	●									
Post-temporal	left							•									
	right						•										
Parietal	left						•	●		•			•				
	right						•	●									
Occipital	left						•	•					•				
	right																

• Rho with p < 0.05 (0.26–0.34); ● rho with p < 0.01 (0.35–0.42); ● rho with p < 0.001 (0.43–0.48); ■ rho with p < 0.0001 (> 0.48). A minus (–) preceding the dot indicates a negative rho.

Table 9/XV. WISC Arithmetic vs 8 s of EEG power (autospectra) while performing mental arithmetic, for the right-preferent sample (n = 56), significant rhos

		Frequency bands															
		1	3	5	7	9	11	13	15	17	19	21	23	25	27	29	31
Prefrontal	left																
	right																
Lat. frontal	left							•					•				
	right											•					
Frontal	left							•		•		•	•				
	right								•	•		•					
Central	left							•		•		●					
	right											•					
Temporal	left					•	•	●	•	•							
	right							•			•	●			•		
Post-temporal	left							•		•							
	right											•					
Parietal	left					•											
	right					•	•										
Occipital	left					•						•					
	right									•							

• Rho with p < 0.05 (0.26–0.34); ● rho with p < 0.01 (0.35–0.42); ● rho with p < 0.001 (0.43–0.48); ■ rho with p < 0.0001 (> 0.48).
A minus (–) preceding the dot indicates a negative rho.

correlates with poor performance in the Comprehension subtest. It appears that the generally observed decrease in EEG activity in patterned Vision is IQ related in the high frequencies, not in the lower.

(2) Table 9/II shows a cluster of negative coefficients, not significant, between 27 and 31 Hz with all coefficients in the 29-Hz band being negative. This negativity of the 29-Hz activity is present in all WISC verbal subtests except Arithmetic and in the WISC performance subtests in Picture Arrangement, Block Design and Object Assembly as well as in the Spatial Relations and Symbol Manipulation tasks from among those developed in our laboratory.

At times the 29-Hz activity is as negative as the 27- and 31-Hz activities (e.g. Analogies and WISC Information). At times the 29-Hz activity is more negative than the neighboring 27 and 31 Hz (as in most of the WISC verbal subtests and especially Digit Span). At times the 29-Hz activity is positive while the 27- and 31-Hz activities are more negative (e.g. WISC Coding, Age and Psychomotor matrices), and finally the 29-Hz activity can be positive, the 27- and 31-Hz activities also being positive (e.g. WISC Arithmetic and Picture Completion).

The 29-Hz activity, even though seldom reaching significance, shows an independence which is surpassed only by the 11- and 13-Hz bands. For the Noise condition, the Comprehension subtests show a column of negative coefficients in the 29-Hz band, one of the few instances in which these negative coefficients reach significance.

For the Noise condition significant negative coefficients are also present from the 27- to 33-Hz bands. It has already been demonstrated [*Giannitrapani,* 1970] that an increase in fast beta activity occurred during the white Noise condition. These significant negative coefficients, which are stronger on the right side, may indicate that during the Noise condition there is a negative relationship between the magnitude of the increase of beta activity on the right side and the scores on the Comprehension subtest. In previous research [*Giannitrapani,* 1971], an increase in beta activity had been postulated as constituting a scanning mechanism, a precursor of the acquisition of meaning. It would be consistent with that finding that in a subject for whom this beta activity occurred to a greater degree the Comprehension score would be low. In other words, greater difficulty in acquiring comprehension is related to a greater amount of beta activity.

Arithmetic

This subtest measures the ability to solve arithmetic story problems. It requires both reasoning and speed of performance, the latter because it is a timed test. Scores, therefore, may be affected by fluctuation of attention as well as motivation. Among the subtests of the Verbal Scale, only Digit Span shows a lower correlation with Verbal IQ.

The Arithmetic subtest, table 9/III, is unique among the verbal subtests in that significant correlations are absent in the lower frequencies, no correlations being significant below the 13-Hz band. The highest correlations are again away from the anterior and posterior poles of the brain and are stronger in general on the left side.

Beyond the cluster from 13 to 17 Hz is a cluster of positive correlations in the 21- to 25-Hz frequency bands. Correlations are lower than in the other cluster, but they are clearly lateralized, left side showing higher coefficients.

It is also of interest to note that the characteristic cluster of negative correlations, which generally occurred in the high beta band in the other verbal subtests, is not present here. This finding points to another major differentiation of the arithmetic function from other verbal functions. Intercorrelation matrices of verbal subtests (table 4/VI) [*Wechsler,* 1949] had clearly indicated the independence of the Arithmetic subtest among the verbal subtests. Given the low level of the correlations and the consequent small amount of variance accounted for, it does not necessarily follow that arithmetic and other verbal functions are inversely related just because the same EEG activity shows positive correlations with the Arithmetic subtest and negative correlations with the other verbal subtests.

Even though individual correlations seldom reach statistical significance, the clustering is definitely significant. Because of the low value of these correlations, it is clear that much of the variance of high beta activity is unaccounted for while a small portion of the variance is inversely related for Arithmetic and the other verbal subtests.

It is also relevant to note that the difficulty in localizing arithmetic functions in the brain is expressed in the present study in the following manner: (1) steady-state EEG correlates with arithmetic performance symmetrically in homologous areas with somewhat higher correlations on the left side (table 9/III) and (2) factor analysis of the EEG obtained while performing mental Arithmetic (fig. 15/5) indicates again primarily bilateral brain involvement with a possible asymmetry favoring right lateral frontal and temporal areas.

The WISC Arithmetic subtest is the only one which is represented in the conditions in which the subjects were administered the EEG. As will be recalled, the fifth condition is mental Arithmetic which consisted of serial subtractions performed in silence with the final answer given aloud. The task is different from the 'story problems' of the WISC subtest, but they both involve mental arithmetic.

It is of interest then to determine what relationships, if any, occur between WISC Arithmetic and brain activity during the 8-second period in which EEG was taken while the subjects were performing mental subtractions. Table 9/XV shows basically the same pattern evident in table 9/III based on the average of all 8 conditions with the addition of a sizeable column of significant positive coefficients in the 21-Hz band.

Inspection of the other individual conditions' matrices (not shown) indicates that WISC Arithmetic is among those intellectual tasks which show great variance in the pattern of significant coefficients with EEG scores. Mental Arithmetic, as well as Resting and Voice, is among those conditions showing greater relationship with WISC Arithmetic.

Similarities

This subtest requires the ability to perceive the common elements between 2 terms. It is regarded as measuring the logical character of the subject's thinking processes as well as the capacity for verbal manipulation. *Wechsler's* intercorrelation matrix (table 4/VI) shows the highest correlations among verbal subtests for Information, Comprehension, Similarities and Vocabulary. When ranking these subtests, while attempting to retain the highest intercorrelation values possible, the Similarities subtest is placed between Comprehension on one hand and Information and Vocabulary on the other. It can be concluded that the Similarities subtest shares with Comprehension a portion of the logical character of the subject's thinking while it shares with Information and Vocabulary a portion of the capacity for verbal manipulation. More of this hierarchy of verbal subtests is to be found in chapter 13.

The Similarities subtest, table 9/IV, shows a pattern of significant correlations very much like the one shown by the Information subtest (table 9/I) but less powerful except for individual correlations in the 13-Hz band. Basically, there is the repetition of a cluster in the central portion of the brain in the 1- to 5-Hz range, a second cluster in the 11- to 13-Hz range (with the notable exception of the prefrontal and occipital areas), the highest correlation being obtained in the left central and right temporal areas (rho = 0.43). There is a small cluster in the frontal and primarily prefrontal areas in the 23- to 27-Hz range, reminiscent of a similar stronger cluster in the Information subtest.

Inspection of individual conditions' matrices (not shown) indicates that the Voice condition has the highest number of positive correlations with WISC Similarities and that the Noise condition has a strong cluster of negative coefficients around the 29-Hz band much like the one obtained for Information under the same EEG condition of listening to white Noise. The cluster in the 23-Hz activity observed in the matrix of the average of all 8 conditions is particularly strong in the Arithmetic and Diffuse vision conditions.

Vocabulary

This subtest requires the subject to define words and, as such, measures the subject's verbal information. It correlates highest with the Information subtest. As with this latter subtest, it relies on the availability of previous funds of knowledge and is least affected by brain damage and age.

The Vocabulary subtest is considered to be one of the best representatives of the verbal battery of the WISC. Table 9/V shows a great similarity between the Vocabulary intercorrelation matrix and that obtained for Comprehension (table 9/II).

There are 3 main clusters: 1–5, 9–13, and 21–23 Hz. The highest correlations are in the 13-Hz band, left and right central areas, rho = 0.51 and 0.47, respectively. The pattern of significant coefficients shown by Vocabulary appears to be representative of the pattern shown by the remaining subtests of the Verbal Scale except for Arithmetic.

Inspection of the individual conditions' matrices (not shown) reveals great similarity among the patterns. The 2 conditions that make the strongest contribution to the average matrix (table 9/V) are those in which the subject was listening to music and to a story, i.e. the 2 patterned auditory conditions. The white Noise matrix shows a cluster of negative correlations similar to that observed when the EEG activity of the same white Noise condition is correlated with WISC Information, Comprehension and Similarities.

Digit Span

This subtest involves the repetition of digits forward and backward and requires intact recent memory and the ability to retain new information. Digits backward is particularly sensitive to attention defects which may be related to difficulties in performing mental tasks requiring sustained concentrated effort. Among the verbal subtests, Digit Span has the smallest correlation with Verbal IQ and among all subtests has the lowest correlation with Full-Scale IQ. *Wechsler* [1944] proposed that the ability involved in Digit Span contains little of the *g* factor, and he quoted *Spearman* as having evidence supporting this.

Parenthetically, the present study shows a right lateralized pattern for this subtest. Performance in this subtest at the high end may be improved by the adoption of strategies such as grouping the digits. Rather than a shortcoming, the capacity for adopting these strategies may be indicative of a capacity for high intellectual function.

This WISC alternate subtest of the Verbal Scale was administered routinely in this study since it was believed to measure an important short-term memory function. Table 9/VI shows for the first time among the subtests of the Verbal Scale a strong occipital component in the 1- and 3-Hz bands. This component is clearly lateralized, favoring the right side, and in the 1-Hz band is significant in the right central area and all posterior areas. There is another cluster of significant positive correlations in frontal, central and temporal areas in the 11- to 15-Hz bands, again stronger on the right side. The highest coefficient is obtained in the right temporal area in the 13-Hz band with a rho = 0.48. There are significant correlations in higher frequency bands as well, in the right prefrontal area (19, 23, and 27 Hz), in the right temporal area (19 and 23 Hz) and in the right post-temporal area (19 Hz). There is only one other WISC verbal subtest which shows higher correlations in the right side, i.e. Information. Among our tests, Symbol Manipulation (table 10/II) also shows higher correlations on the right side. While both Digit Span and Symbol Manipulation involve dealing with numerical sequences and short-term memory for sequences, the relationship with Information is less clear.

Inspection of individual conditions (not shown) indicates considerable independence between matrices. The 13-Hz cluster of significant coefficients is present throughout except for Arithmetic where the 11- and 19-Hz components as well as the prefrontal and temporal components are observable.

The strongest conditions for Digit Span are the 2 visual conditions in which a great deal of significant frequency related activity is present (11–27 Hz) as well as brain-areas related activity, particularly right temporal.

Picture Completion

This subtest requires the subject to discover the missing part of a picture, and it measures the ability to recognize missing details in familiar objects. It also requires an internal search for relevant details.

Table 9/VII shows the first intercorrelation matrix of the subtests of the Performance Scale. There are several significant coefficients in the 1-Hz band as well as in the 13-Hz band. In addition to these 2 clusters, there is a cluster of significant coefficients in a broad range of beta frequencies from 19 to 31 Hz in the prefrontal areas, primarily on the left side. This pattern is reminiscent of the one observed in the Information and Similarities subtests. They are the only ones showing left prefrontal significant coefficients for beta activity. The only other prefrontal finding is on the right side in the Digit Span subtest.

The left occipital component is not very strong here, but it will be noted to a greater or lesser extent in all performance subtests as well as Arithmetic. It will be remembered that among the verbal subtests there appeared a cluster of negative coefficients in the high beta frequencies which at times reached significance. No such cluster is observable in this performance subtest pooled matrix, while inspection of individual subtest matrices (not shown) reveals a strong though not significant cluster of high beta activity for the Voice condition.

The prefrontal component of positive significant coefficients in beta frequencies is strongest in the Music condition. The beta negativity characteristic of the subtests of the Verbal Scale is present during Voice, a verbal auditory task, while positive beta coefficients, a nonverbal characteristic, occur to a greater degree during Music, a nonverbal task. Also to be noted is a left occipital component which appears, in addition to the average matrix, in the Music, Voice and Arithmetic conditions. Great variance among individual conditions' matrices is shown for this subtest. In the mental Arithmetic condition, e.g. this is observable in figures 5/2, 5/3 and 5/4. For the 11-Hz band (fig. 5/2), to be noted is the fact that a particularly high number of significant correlations is present among the cross-spectra with the exclusion of significant correlations among the autospectra. This particular dimension (the meaning of the differential between the relationships obtained with autospectra and cross-spectra) has not yet been studied.

Picture Arrangement

This subtest requires the subject to rearrange a series of pictures in order to convey a meaningful story. It measures a subject's ability to comprehend and size-up the total situation. *Wechsler* [1944] did not believe that it measures 'social intelligence'. He held that social intelligence is not a separate entity but is simply general intelligence applied to social situations. While this may be a purely semantic argument, the present research indicates some very specific EEG features related to the scores of this subtest. The present investigator holds that there is great individual difference in the manner that people are sensitive to social nuances, and whether this is a personality trait or not, the independence of the picture arrangement scores from the Full-Scale IQ scores indicates that this subtest is measuring a relatively independent function.

In table 9/VIII there begins to emerge a pattern, typical of some of the subtests of the Performance Scale, of negative coefficients in the theta frequency band. In this subtest some of the negative coefficients in the 5- and 7-Hz bands actually reach significance. Perhaps this phenomenon is due to imperfect age-scaling norms in the subtests showing this pattern. It may indicate, however, an inverse relationship between theta activity and ability to deal with circumstances in the present surroundings which is one of the major underlying prerequisites for good performance in the Picture Arrangement subtest.

In terms of lateralization of functions, *Reitan* [1955] and *Meier and French* [1966] have shown with right anterior temporal lesions a rather specific deficit in the Picture Arrangement subtest. In the matrix of EEG relationships discussed here (table 9/VIII), the anterior temporal region would be represented by the lateral frontal placement surrounded by the prefrontal, frontal and temporal placements. The matrix of table 9/VIII shows that the lateral frontal, frontal and temporal placements have a greater number of correlations, higher even though not significant, on the right side. It would be erroneous to conclude, however, that the right hemisphere presides over all the functions subsumed under the Picture Arrangements subtest.

There is also a broad cluster of significant positive coefficients of beta activity from 13 to 23 Hz from central to occipital areas with clear lateralization in the left central and left occipital areas. This cluster is vaguely reminiscent of the pattern of significant coefficients shown by the Symbol Manipulation test developed in our laboratory (table 10/II) and the WISC Arithmetic subtest (table 9/III). The major difference between the latter and Picture Arrangement is that in Arithmetic significance is shown also in more anterior areas.

Inspection of the individual conditions' matrices (not shown) reveals great variance but a persistence of essentially the central and occipital components. For instance, there may be observed during Music a potentiated cluster of the low frequency negative coefficients as well as the retention of the 17-Hz component.

While performing mental Arithmetic, instead, the low frequency negative component does not reach significance, but all frequencies above 11 Hz (except 29 Hz) are represented as well as the left central and left occipital areas as shown in the average matrix of table 9/VIII. The left occipital component is also observed in Arithmetic as well as in all the Performance subtests to a greater or lesser degree.

Block Design

This subtest requires the subject to reproduce with blocks a geometrical design furnished by a test figure. It requires the ability to analyze a gestalt, breaking it into its components and reconstructing it. Among the subtests of the Performance Scale it is the one having strongest correlation with Verbal IQ and Full-Scale IQ.

Wechsler (table 4/VI) demonstrated that Block Design, among the subtests of the Performance Scale, has the highest correlation with subtests of the Verbal Scale. The pattern shown in table 9/IX bears out this relationship insofar that the significant correlations are reminiscent of those obtained in the Comprehension subtest. There are 3 clusters: the first from 1 to 7 Hz, the second from 11 to 17 Hz and the third from 23 to 25 Hz. The findings are lateralized with, in general, higher coefficients on the left side.

Inspection of the individual subtests' matrices (not shown) reveals basically the same pattern, the white Noise condition showing the lowest coefficients and Arithmetic the highest. While the left occipital component does not stand out above others in this matrix, it should be noted that it occurs, as mentioned earlier, in Arithmetic and in all other performance subtests.

Object Assembly

This subtest consists of a series of figure formboards to be reassembled so as to form familiar figures. Among all of the subtests, Object Assembly correlates least with Verbal IQ and most with Performance IQ. This subtest, table 9/X, shows as in the Picture Arrangement subtest a strong pattern of negative coefficients in a broad range of frequencies without, however, reaching significance. Significant coefficients are very rare, only in the 13- and 23-Hz bands, and are stronger on the left side. Even though there is a minimal left occipital significant component, the latter acquires dominant proportion in some of the conditions (e.g. Voice not shown). The low relationship between EEG scores and this subtest reflects the low correlation found by *Wechsler* (table 4/VI) between this subtest and all other WISC subtests. Wechsler's intercorrelation matrix shows that this performance subtest is the best single representative of Performance IQ, having the highest correlation among all subtests with Performance IQ. Wechsler's matrix also shows object assembly as having the lowest correlations among those obtained between performance subtests and verbal subtests.

These features of Wechsler's intercorrelation pattern in conjunction with the fact that for this subtest the fewest correlations with EEG scores are obtained reemphasize that the EEG autospectra parameters studied in this investigation are least sensitive to the performance variables studied. The EEG cross spectra parameters, e.g. figures 5/2, 5/3, and 5/4, also show a similar low incidence of correlations with Object Assembly. It seems that we have not yet located the most sensitive frequency range nor the most sensitive EEG parameters for the study of performance variables.

Coding

This subtest requires the subject to substitute a series of digits with the symbols to be found in the given key. It constitutes a measure of visuomotor functioning.

Table 9/XI shows a relatively high number of negative correlations (not reaching significance). The negative coefficients in the low frequency spectra were interpreted in chapter 4 in the discussion of table 4/I as representing an inverse relationship between random eye movements and purposeful eye movements, a necessary requisite for successful performance in this timed subtest. The cluster of negative correlations in the Coding subtest is different from that obtained in Picture Arrangement in that for the former the negative correlations are higher in a lower frequency range. This fact is consistent with the hypothesis that the performance in coding is affected by eye movements of the subject. In spectral analysis, artifacts of eye movements cluster in the 1- to 5-Hz range and in anterior parasagittal areas.

Positive coefficients in the left occipital area characteristic of the performance subtests are a unique feature here. This occipital pattern is rather stable and is found to be strongest in the Voice condition (not shown).

It seems reasonable to conclude that while most of the other subtests (especially the verbal ones) involve several brain areas and therefore measure more complex functions, Coding measures a unitary function of visual search and processing of information which correlates with the presence of several frequencies of EEG activity in the occipital areas, primarily on the left side.

Verbal IQ

The first summary score of the WISC in table 9/XII shows basically the pattern of the Comprehension subtest with some minor changes and the increase in coefficients, especially in the 11- and 13-Hz bands, the latter being a strong component in all of the verbal subtests. The highest coefficients are in the left and right central areas and in the right temporal area of the 13-Hz band with a rho = 0.50 for all 3 areas. There is not a clear lateralization pattern in this composite score.

Inspection of the individual conditions' matrices (not shown) reveals basically the same pattern of significance in most brain areas except the occipitals. The Noise condition should be mentioned because in that matrix the negative 29-Hz activity as well as other negative high beta activity acquires considerable significance.

Performance IQ

It was obvious from the inspection of the performance subtests' matrices that fewer significant coefficients occurred between the EEG scores and values on the performance subtests compared with the corresponding coefficients on the verbal subtests. The pattern shown by the Performance IQ (table 9/XIII) indicates that in general there is very little activity in the basal EEG that has either a direct or inverse relationship with the ability necessary for carrying out tasks involved in Performance IQ. This table shows a small cluster in the 13-Hz band and activity in the left occipital area from the 13- to 25-Hz bands with highest correlations being rho = 0.39 in the 13-Hz band for the left central area and in the 23-Hz band for the left occipital area.

Inspection of individual conditions' subtests reveals greater disparity in the patterns than that obtained for the verbal subtests. This feature is also observed among the individual conditions' matrices for Performance IQ as compared with the individual conditions' matrices for Verbal IQ (not shown). The matrix for patterned Vision, for instance, shows a few scattered negative coefficients.

The matrix for mental Arithmetic shows strong 11-, 13-, 23-, and 25-Hz activity in most leads except the most anterior, while the Voice condition shows a pattern very similar to the overall pattern for Performance IQ. The lower correlations in Performance IQ may be responsible for this lower reliability of given EEG conditions in predicting intellectual performance, but there is definite evidence that EEG amplitude contains features that are more sensitive to different aspects of Verbal IQ.

Full-Scale IQ

This overall score of the WISC, table 9/XIV, retains a strong 11-Hz component but an even stronger 13-Hz component. Since significant coefficients in the 13-Hz band appeared in most of the verbal and some of the performance subtests, this composite score reflected coefficients which are the highest obtained among all the subtests, reaching a value of + 0.60 in the left central area.

It is not understood at this point why such a relatively small amount of EEG activity in the occipital and prefrontal areas was related to intellectual functioning as measured by the WISC. Another question is why the central areas and in particular the left central area, time and again, seem to carry the largest portion of activity which was positively related to the intellectual functions tested.

In the 23-Hz band there is a scatter of significant correlations among all brain areas, primarily on the left side. It is of interest to note that for Verbal IQ in this frequency the significant coefficients were in the anterior areas while for Performance IQ they were in the posterior areas. Inspection of individual subtest matrices indicates that most of the verbal subtests had a 23-Hz component while for the performance subtests only the Block Design had a relatively large number of significant correlations in this frequency band.

Inspection of individual conditions' matrices (not shown) reveals a basic stability of the 11- and 13-Hz components which were present in both verbal and performance subtests and greater variability in the other frequencies. The lowest number of significant coefficients was obtained for the Noise condition while Voice was among the highest. No coefficient among those of the individual conditions' matrices reached the level of + 0.60 obtained for Full-Scale IQ and pooled conditions in the left central area.

References

Giannitrapani, D.: EEG changes under differing auditory stimulations. Archs gen. Psychiat. *23:* 445–453 (1970).

Giannitrapani, D.: Scanning mechanisms and the EEG. Electroenceph. clin. Neurophysiol. *30:* 139–146 (1971).

Giannitrapani, D.: The electroencephalogram of mental abilities; in Wilkinson, Investigation of brain function, pp. 35–58 (Plenum Publishing, New York 1981).

Meier, M.J.; French, L.A.: Longitudinal assessment of intellectual function following unilateral temporal lobectomy. J. clin. Psychol. *22:* 22 (1966).

Reitan, R.M.: Certain differential effects of left and right cerebral lesions in human adults. J. compar. physiol. Psychol. *48:* 474–477 (1955).

Wechsler, D.: The measurement of adult intelligence; 3rd ed. (Williams & Wilkins, Baltimore 1944).

Wechsler, D.: WISC manual, Wechsler Intelligence Scale for Children (Psychological Corp., New York 1949).

10 Other Intellectual Variables

'The scientific method, as far as it is a method, is nothing more than doing one's damnedest with one's mind, no holds barred.'
P.W. Bridgman

Spatial Relations

Age norms were not available for this test which was developed at the laboratory. The scores are raw scores not corrected for age. Table 10/I shows remarkably few significant correlations. Those present are of low significance. There is a tendency to interpret these correlations as constituting a random phenomenon except perhaps for the small cluster in the central areas in the 13-Hz band.

Subdivision of this matrix into the individual conditions' matrices (not shown) indicates few notable features such as significant positive coefficients in the 13-Hz band except for the 2 visual conditions and overwhelmingly negative coefficients in the 29-Hz band.

Findings indicate that the presence of 13-Hz activity (which this research has shown to have a strong verbal component) is mildly related to the performance of Spatial Relations. The fact that this relationship does not reach statistical significance in the 2 visual conditions is perhaps a resultant of the decrease of activity in that frequency when the subject has eyes open.

Symbol Manipulation

This lingual nonverbal test was also developed at the laboratory, and the scores are in raw form. In table 10/II we begin to see the development of the 11- to 13-Hz activity as well as of the higher frequencies with an asymmetrical pattern appearing among homologous areas, the right side showing higher positive correlations. There is also a cluster of significant negative correlations appearing in high beta frequencies in the left temporal area. Occipital areas are clearly involved.

Subdivision into conditions' matrices (not shown) indicates in general that the same occipital pattern is observable in all conditions except mental Arithmetic and that there is a relatively strong 19- and 21-Hz component that is positively related to this activity. The overwhelming majority of the significant coefficients among the frequencies of 23 Hz and above is negative, highest values being in general in the temporal and especially left temporal areas.

It seems that this Symbol Manipulation task, verbal in nature, is performed via visual as well as auditory processes if one can make an inference from the clustering of significant coefficients (whether positive or negative) in the occipital and temporal areas.

Verbal Analogies

Age norms were not available for the Analogies test, also developed at the laboratory. Table 10/III shows a similarity to the Symbol Manipulation test, namely the clustering of significant correlations in the 11- and 13-Hz bands, the homologous asymmetries with higher correlations on the right side, the highest positive correlation in the right temporal area and the cluster of negative correlations in the high beta range of the left temporal area. There is more anterior activity involved here than in the Symbol Manipulation task, but the latter obtained stronger positive correlations and in a broader range of frequencies.

The negative cluster of coefficients of beta activity in the left temporal area is of particular interest. It will be remembered that there is a negative correlation of beta activity with age and that the left temporal region contributed very little significance to this cluster. The existence of significant negative correlations in this brain area for this task cannot be related to age. These findings demonstrate that the presence of fast beta activity in the left temporal area is not wholly related to the presence of the same activity in other parts of the brain nor in the homologous right temporal area.

The data also indicate that Analogies are positively related to the presence of 11- and 13-Hz activity in most brain areas, especially on the right side, while they are negatively related to the presence of fast beta activity in the left temporal area.

Inspection of the coefficients obtained for the individual EEG conditions (not shown) indicates that the Analogies task is among those with the greatest differences in significant coefficients among conditions, but the higher negative coefficients of beta activity in the left temporal area are

Table 10/I. Spatial relations vs 64 s of EEG power (autospectra) for the right-preferent sample (n = 56), significant rhos

		Frequency bands															
		1	3	5	7	9	11	13	15	17	19	21	23	25	27	29	31
Prefrontal	left																
	right																
Lat. frontal	left															−•	
	right																
Frontal	left												•				
	right			•				•									
Central	left							•									
	right							•									
Temporal	left															−•	
	right																
Post-temporal	left																
	right																
Parietal	left												•				
	right																
Occipital	left																
	right																

• Rho with p < 0.05 (0.26–0.34); ● rho with p < 0.01 (0.35–0.42); ● rho with p < 0.001 (0.43–0.48); ■ rho with p < 0.0001 (> 0.48).
A minus (–) preceding the dot indicates a negative rho.

Table 10/II. Symbol manipulation vs 64 s of EEG power (autospectra) for the right-preferent sample (n = 56), significant rhos

		Frequency bands															
		1	3	5	7	9	11	13	15	17	19	21	23	25	27	29	31
Prefrontal	left																
	right																
Lat. frontal	left																
	right																
Frontal	left																
	right							•	•								
Central	left							●									
	right							●									
Temporal	left							●						−•	−•	−•		−•
	right						●	●	•								
Post-temporal	left							•									
	right						•	•		•	●						
Parietal	left																
	right						•	•		•							
Occipital	left						•										
	right						•	•		•	●	•					

• Rho with p < 0.05 (0.26–0.34); ● rho with p < 0.01 (0.35–0.42); ● rho with p < 0.001 (0.43–0.48); ■ rho with p < 0.0001 (> 0.48).
A minus (–) preceding the dot indicates a negative rho.

present throughout even though not always reaching significance. They are particularly strong in the Voice, the patterned Vision and the Diffuse vision conditions and are strongest in the latter. The Diffuse vision condition (not shown) is the most significant representative of table 10/III, having some correlations even stronger than those shown in the table.

The mental Arithmetic condition is the least representative of table 10/III with none of the mentioned clusters present but with a significant positive cluster in the right lateral frontal for frequency bands 19–25, a significant positive cluster in the right temporal for frequency bands 9–13, and a considerable number of negative coefficients in the 1- and 3-Hz band primarily in temporal and posterior areas, significant on the left side.

Psychomotor Efficiency

The last of the tests generated at the laboratory is in raw score form, not corrected for age. It will be recalled that it consists of rapidly checking groups of digits for identity or diversity. Rapid, efficient visual scanning is required, with a visual memory for rows of digits being helpful. It is not necessarily an intellectual task by a narrow definition of the term, but it was included here because it represented what was believed to be an important function in the processing of information, i.e. the ability to scan efficiently and arrive quickly at a decision. This task was believed to measure an important aspect of the efficiency with which the brain executed input and output functions.

Table 10/IV shows a whole array of negative correlations. It is the only measure with overwhelmingly negative correlations except age.

Two possibilities arise: (1) These correlations may be a function of an age-related phenomenon, namely that this psychomotor facility develops perceivably with age, at least among 11- to 13-year-olds. (2) The other alternative, and the 2 alternatives are not necessarily mutually exclusive, is that the presence of 1- to 7-Hz activity hinders efficient visual scanning and processing of information.

Inspection of the individual conditions (not shown) reveals basically the same pattern with, in addition, a cluster of significant positive correlations in the occipital areas during the Voice condition. This difference indicates that while listening to a story there is an increase in the 13-Hz activity in the occipital areas and that this increase is positively related to the performance of the Psychomotor task.

Table 10/III. Verbal analogies vs 64 s of EEG power (autospectra) for the right-preferent sample (n = 56), significant rhos

		Frequency bands														
		1	3	5	7	9	11	13	15	17	19	21	23	25	27	29	31
Prefrontal	left						•										
	right						•										
Lat. frontal	left																
	right						•	•			•						
Frontal	left						•										
	right						•	•									
Central	left						•	•									
	right						•	•									
Temporal	left							•						−•	−•	−•	−•
	right						•	●									
Post-temporal	left						•	•									
	right						•	•			•						
Parietal	left							•									
	right						•	●									
Occipital	left																
	right						•										

• Rho with p < 0.05 (0.26–0.34); ● rho with p < 0.01 (0.35–0.42); ● rho with p < 0.001 (0.43–0.48); ■ rho with p < 0.0001 (> 0.48).
A minus (–) preceding the dot indicates a negative rho.

Table 10/IV. Psychomotor efficiency vs 64 s of EEG power (autospectra) for the right-preferent sample (n = 56), significant rhos

		Frequency bands														
		1	3	5	7	9	11	13	15	17	19	21	23	25	27	29	31
Prefrontal	left																
	right																
Lat. frontal	left		−•	−●													
	right			−•													
Frontal	left		−●	−•										−•			
	right		−●	−•													
Central	left	−•	−●	−●	−•												
	right		−●	−●													
Temporal	left		−●	−●	−•						−•				−•		
	right		−•	−●	−•												
Post-temporal	left	−•	−●	−•											−•		−●
	right		−•	−•													
Parietal	left	−•	−●	−•													
	right		−●	−•												•	
Occipital	left																
	right																

• Rho with p < 0.05 (0.26–0.34); ● rho with p < 0.01 (0.35–0.42); ● rho with p < 0.001 (0.43–0.48); ■ rho with p < 0.0001 (> 0.48).
A minus (–) preceding the dot indicates a negative rho.

11 Functional Role of Brain Areas

'It is proposed that the self-conscious mind plays through the whole liaison brain in a selective and unifying manner ... Perhaps ... some multiple scanning and probing device that reads out from and selects from the immense and diverse patterns of activity in the liaison brain and integrates these selected components, so organizing them into the unity of conscious experience.'
Sir *John Eccles*

This chapter will discuss the functional role of each brain area tested, based upon the interpretation of the significant rhos presented in the matrices of correlations between EEG and intellectual variables in chapters 9 and 10.

Frontal Poles

The EEG data from the prefrontal leads was obtained according to the 10–20 system from Fp_1 and Fp_2 placements, basically from electrodes placed 1 inch above the supraorbital arch above the center of the orbits. Unfortunately, the dream of finding strong evidence for the intellectual role of the prefrontal brain areas has again been shattered. The data of the present study shows that these areas are among those having the smallest number of significant correlations with intellectual scores but that these areas serve some intellectual functions not served primarily by other brain areas nor by more posterior areas of the frontal lobes.

Of the significant correlations obtained, only one is retained for Full-Scale IQ (table 9/XIV) in the Fp_1 for the 23-Hz activity and none for Performance IQ (table 9/XIII). Among the performance subtests the only significant correlations are in the Picture Completion subtest in a span from 18 to 32 Hz primarily on the left side. This pattern, the strongest for any of the subtests, is reminiscent of the findings of *Cohen* [1957a, b] in his factor analysis of the Wechsler Adult Intelligence Scale (WAIS). Cohen found that the Picture Completion subtest had a specificity of its own extractable as a separate factor with few other loadings.

But, what may this factor be? *Pribram* [1959], working with monkeys, concluded: 'Frontal intrinsic sector lesions interfere with those aspects of intention that depend on an estimation of the effects that an outcome has in terms of the total set of possible outcomes that are available.' While this proposition could hold for Block Design as well, the fundamental difference between the 2 subtests is that in the latter the task is to duplicate an end product which is given, while in the former the product must be found among an array of possibilities from within the subject's experiences. It is perhaps the same difference that exists between a multiple choice question and one with a blank for a word to be filled in by the subject.

Luria [1969] summarized the lateralization of frontal-lobe findings as follows: '...intellectual operations demand(ing) the creation of a program of action and a choice between several equally probable alternatives... are seen particularly clearly in patients with bilateral lesions of the frontal lobes or with massive lesions of the frontal lobe of the dominant (left) hemisphere, and they may be hardly demonstrable in patients with a lesion of the right frontal lobe or of the orbital portions of the frontal cortex.'

Among the subtests of the verbal scale, this *furnished-from-within* quality is shared in different degrees by Information, Comprehension and Similarities, all having some significant correlations with EEG power in the prefrontal areas (tables 9/I, 9/II, 9/IV).

Another deficit with frontal pole lesions, originally observed by *Malmo* [1942], is in the responses requiring a certain delay [*Luria*, 1969]. It seems that in these cases what is lacking is a certain facility in handling short-term memory. The fact that the Digit Span subtest (table 9/VI) shows significant correlations with the right frontal pole is possibly related to that. It appears that judging the appropriateness of certain responses is dependent upon the presence of certain EEG frequencies primarily in the left frontal pole, while the activity of the right frontal pole is more related to certain aspects of short-term memory.

The work of *Stamm and Rosen* [1973] is of interest in discussing this role of the right frontal pole. In working with monkeys with intact frontal lobes and using a stimulation technique, delayed response performance was found to be altered by unilateral stimulus application to prefrontal areas of the cortex contralateral to the preferred hand. These alterations could occur either on the left or right side but contralateral to the hand with which the monkey had received extensive training.

The correlations with Digit Span (table 9/VI) in the present experiment are unilateral, but ipsilateral to the preferred hand. It could be that phylogenetically this function was replaced in the dominant hemisphere by the more abstract portion of this function, i.e. the capacity for sorting out relevant details. The more concrete aspects of this function, i.e. the ability to resist the intrusion of irrelevant material was retained in man in a relatively minor role and migrated to the homologous prefrontal area of the nondominant hemisphere.

Luria [1966], in summarizing deficits ascertained by injuries to the orbital part of the frontal cortex, indicated that perhaps because of the close connection of these areas with the limbic system, the main characteristics of the syndrome shift toward affective disorders. While the present investigation was not directed at studying affective systems, the primary set of correlations observed in these areas indicates that a role in intellectual functions is served by the prefrontal areas which is not served primarily by other brain areas nor by more posterior areas of the frontal lobes.

A portion of the frontal lobe syndrome diffusely attributed to damage of large frontal lobe areas seems to be relegated by this technique to prefrontal areas. More specifically, *Luria* [1966] described the deficits as '...an inability to remain within the limits of the selective system of connections given by the text, a ready emergence of irrelevant connections and an inability to inhibit these irrelevant connections'.

The correlations found between EEG activity of the left prefrontal area and Picture Completion (table 9/VII) could very well constitute a correlate of the facility for abstracting the relevant missing portion of the figure among the many possible alternatives available to the subject. Furthermore, the correlations found in the right prefrontal area with Digit Span may indicate that the right prefrontal area is more concerned with the not-quite-verbal aspect of the delayed reaction deficit – a deficit which would certainly affect the logical sequence of responses and which is usually not separated from the damage to abstract thinking.

Lateral Frontal Areas

The electrode placements for the study of these areas were F_7 and F_8 of the 10–20 system, approximately half way between the frontal and the temporal placements (1 inch above the preauricular point) on the coronal plane.

This placement is regarded to be usually in a location anterior to Broca's area and occasionally to occur on or near the Sylvian fissure.

The Full-Scale IQ matrix (table 9/XIV) indicates significant correlations in alpha bands from 10 to 14 Hz. This is clearly due to the contributions of the Verbal IQ component (table 9/XII) because no such relationship is present in the Performance IQ matrix (table 9/XIII).

This lack of correlations between the EEG activity of those brain areas and Performance IQ holds through all performance subtests with two small exceptions. One is Block Design (table 9/IX) with significant correlations on the left side in the 13- and 23-Hz bands, and the other is Picture Arrangement (table 9/VIII) with significant negative correlations in the 5- and 7-Hz bands bilaterally. In both subtests these correlations are not a component of the main cluster of significant correlations for those subtests but are perhaps an indicator of some minor role served by these areas in the performance of those tasks. In the case of Block Design these left-sided correlations may be an indicator of one of the verbal functions needed for the performance of that task as reinforced by the unilateral correlations of the frontal areas to be discussed in the next section (Mid-Frontal Areas).

The Picture Arrangement negative correlations from 4 to 8 Hz are among the rare instances in which intellectual variables were negatively related to EEG power, indicating that a decrease of 4- to 8-Hz activity was related to better scores on the Picture Arrangement subtest.

One of the possibilities is that this relationship is the resultant of an age-related artifact. It could be postulated that the presence of theta activity as an expression of emotional involvement [*Walter,* 1950, 1953] might hamper a cool and dispassionate evaluation of the possible sequences in the Picture Arrangement subtest. One could not discount the possibility, however, that the different maturational processes involved in the solution of Picture Arrangement have different maturational rates and that the weighted score on this subtest corrected for the average of these maturational processes. The matrix of correlations in table 9/VIII permitted the study of the different components of this task separately. The lateral frontal component of the task may have a maturational rate not completely corrected by the pragmatic normalization of the Wechsler Intelligence Scale for Children (WISC). Another rationale for these negative correlations is that they may be consequent to eye-movement artifacts (cf. discussion of type 3 factors in chapter 12).

These lateral frontal areas, however, show greater relationship with verbal subtests. While we are not dealing yet with the areas which show the

greatest overall verbal relationship as shown for the mid-frontal relationship for Verbal IQ (table 9/XII), the following relationships are found
among the individual verbal subtests.

While Information, Arithmetic, Similarities and Digit Span show some
relationship with alpha power, correlations are more numerous for Vocabulary, the most solid band of correlations occurring with alpha activity from
8 to 14 Hz bilaterally. In addition to alpha activity, Comprehension (table
9/II) shows left-sided correlations in the 7- and 23-Hz bands, frequencies
whose relationships with this subtest shall recur in other brain areas.

From the above analysis and from an analysis of the existing literature
on the functions of these areas, it is difficult to attribute a very specific
function to these areas except for a very general verbal role primarily
mediated by a broad alpha band. Among the performance subtests the pattern of correlations for the Block Design subtest is similar to those of the
Comprehension subtest but reaches significance only twice on the left side
in the 13- and 23-Hz bands. This emphasizes the similarity of Block Design
to verbal subtests, a similarity which had been observed in the original
WISC subtests intercorrelation matrix (table 4/VI). Block Design correlates
higher with verbal subtests than any of the other performance subtests.
Additional discussion of the functional role of these areas is to be found in
chapters 15 and 16.

Mid-Frontal Areas

The mid-frontal placements (FL, FR) were obtained by trisecting the
distance between F_7 and F_8. In reference to the 10–20 system FL is between
F_z and F_3 near F_3 while FR is between F_z and F_4 near F_4.

The mid-frontal areas show the greatest number of significant correlations with Full-Scale IQ (table 9/XIV), clearly involving a broad range of
frequencies from 4 to 24 Hz. Again the Performance IQ table is noncon-
tributing while in the Verbal IQ matrix (table 9/XII) the correlations reach
higher levels in general and reach significance in a practically unbroken frequency span from 0 to 26 Hz. The individual performance subtests which do
show significant correlations are: (1) Picture Completion (table 9/VII) with a
pattern seemingly related to the fast beta activity (27- and 31-Hz bands)
present in the adjacent prefrontal areas; (2) Block Design (table 9/IX) with a
broad range of frequencies clearly left-lateralized, reminiscent of the pattern
obtained for Verbal IQ; and (3) Coding (table 9/XI) with negative correla-

tions for the 3-Hz band bilaterally which seems to be determined by eye-movement artifacts and which was interpreted in chapters 4, 5 and 9.

All verbal subtests except Digit Span show the largest number of significant correlations with the EEG frequencies of these areas indicating, according to these measurements, a verbal role even greater than the role of the temporal areas. The subtest with the largest number of significant correlations in these areas is Comprehension with a relatively symmetrical bilateral role in processing verbal abstractions.

Digit Span (table 9/VI) retains significance only in the 13-Hz band bilaterally, the subtest obviously not involving abstract functions.

A summary of the frontal areas anterior to sensory-motor functions follows: apparently the mid-frontal areas serve a multiple bilaterally integrative function of abstract verbal material. This function must be different from the relatively minor left-lateralized verbal function presided over by the lateral frontal area which may serve to elaborate the material originating in Broca's area. Different again is the role of the prefrontal areas which, even though primarily verbal, show on each side two different aspects of a function which seems to relate to a capacity for focusing and resistance to intrusion of unrelated stimuli.

It is possible now to review and more precisely localize the different descriptions of deficits observed by different authors in regard to frontal lobe lesions. *Denny-Brown's* [1951] inability to behave in accordance with plans, *Luria's* [1966] movements which fall under the influence of irrelevant factors, *Freeman and Watts'* [1942] distortion of awareness of the self and of one's actions, and *Malmo's* [1948] inability to maintain the stable purpose of behavior would all be mediated primarily by the prefrontal areas, while *Goldstein's* [1936] disturbance of abstract attitude and categorical thinking, and *Brickner's* [1936] disturbance of the synthesis of engrams would result from disturbance in the mid-frontal functions. One should not, however, conclude from this that the processing of verbal material is restricted to the frontal areas. Further analysis will demonstrate the wide utilization of brain areas for mediating such complex functions.

Central Areas

The central placements (CL, CR) were obtained by trisecting the distance between T_3 and T_4 on a frontal plane. In reference to the 10–20 system CL is between C_z and C_3 near C_3 while CR is between C_z and C_4

near C_4. Anatomically these electrodes are near the sensory-motor areas, most probably in a placement anterior to the precentral gyrus.

These areas show again a heavy loading in verbal areas. Full-Scale IQ (table 9/XIV) shows, after the mid-frontal areas, the largest number of significant correlations. The highest rho for the matrix is also here, 0.60 in the left central area for the 13-Hz band, while for the other frequencies correlations are generally higher on the right side.

While Performance IQ shows significance only in the 13-Hz band, Verbal IQ shows a pattern similar to Full-Scale IQ except that for the former there is a left-sided lateralization. The pattern found in Performance IQ for this area is representative of the Picture Completion and the Object Assembly subtests, and for the latter constitutes together with the left temporal area the only cluster of significance. Block Design presents a picture very similar to Verbal IQ with perhaps more emphasis on the right side, while Picture Arrangement shows a unique pattern. There is significance in the ubiquitous 13-Hz band and in addition in the 15- and 17-Hz bands, the latter also showing significant clusters only for Block Design and Arithmetic.

Among the verbal subtests Coding is noncontributory and Digit Span shows a pattern similar to Performance IQ. Information and Similarities show significance in the very low frequencies and in the 11- and 13-Hz bands. This pattern gathers momentum in Vocabulary with the addition of significance in the 9- and 23-Hz bands and in Comprehension with the further addition of the 15- and 21-Hz bands. Arithmetic presents a different picture with a cluster of significance between 12 and 18 Hz.

In summary, while these areas seem to serve a primarily verbal function with a small degree of lateralization, if any, the activity in the 13-Hz band is common to performance functions as well. It would be interesting to determine whether the relationship between 13-Hz activity and performance functions is not really due to a verbal component of performance tasks which might be absent or minimal in the Coding subtest (cf. chapter 12).

One can assume that the placement of these electrodes is in the neighborhood of the premotor system, in which case *Luria's* [1966] summary is pertinent. He concluded that the specific intellectual deficits related to lesions of these areas are disturbances in the dynamics of the intellectual process and more specifically in the inability to synthesize and automate habitual mental actions.

Because of the ubiquity of this process all subtests (except Coding) show an effect, and as mentioned before, the highest correlation with Full-Scale IQ is found in this area in the 13-Hz band. The fact that the Coding subtest is particularly excluded from any relevance to this process (the correlations obtained for 13-Hz activity in the 2 central areas are 0.06 and 0.07, respectively) leads to the inference that the automation referred to above is for more abstract mental operations than those required while 'coding'.

One could then form a subtest hierarchy based on the relative presence of this synthesizing function – as inferred from the significance of the rhos between 13-Hz activity in the central areas and specific subtests. Casting aside Coding, the progression would be as follows: Digit Span, Object Assembly, Picture Completion, Similarities (which can be solved via concrete processes), Information, Block Design, Vocabulary and finally Comprehension. Arithmetic and Picture Arrangement are differentiated from the above group because of relationships in the 17-Hz band which will be discussed further in chapter 12. This hierarchy pertains to component functions assumed to be specifically served by the central areas, and it is not in contradiction with the regional hierarchy of WISC subtests proposed in chapter 13.

Temporal Areas

The temporal placements T_3, T_4 correspond approximately to a position 1 inch above the pre-auricular point. The complexity of the different roles of these areas is badly represented by the apparently simple pattern shown by the Full-Scale IQ matrix. Significance is found in the 11- and 13-Hz bands bilaterally and in a unique negative correlation in the 29-Hz band on the left side. Among the subtests, this latter correlation is found only in Information, but the specific role and patterning of the 29-Hz activity is discussed in the section dealing with that frequency.

Performance IQ (table 9/XIII) shows only a left-sided significant rho in the 13-Hz band, and while Verbal IQ shows a broad band of right-sided correlations from 0 to 14 Hz, Verbal IQ again shows the largest number of relationships. Unexpected was the lateralization of the verbal material in the nondominant side.

Among the performance subtests, the left lateralization is reproduced in the Block Design and Object Assembly subtests while Picture Arrangement seemed to right-lateralize in faster frequencies (15 and 19 Hz). In Picture Completion the positive relationship with slow delta activity (1-Hz band) is difficult to interpret at this time.

Among the verbal subtests, Comprehension is the strongest contributor of left-sided correlations (from 0 to 14 Hz), while Digit Span is the strongest contributor of right-sided rhos (from 10 to 24 Hz). Information, Similarities and Vocabulary show, on the right side, the same general pattern shown by Comprehension on the left side, while Arithmetic continues the pattern shown in other areas of significant rhos in a band from 12 to 18 Hz. The diversity in frequencies and in the pattern of lateralization of these areas is among the largest observed in these matrices.

The pattern of significance for the different intellectual measures is quite diverse and somewhat baffling. The findings are primarily on the right side and the literature is very skimpy in this regard. *Luria* [1966], in discussing disturbances of higher cortical functions with temporal lesions, mentioned the paucity of studies dealing with right-sided lesions and limited himself to presenting evidence for left-sided findings, i.e. deficits in mental arithmetic, in the phonemic and conceptual structure of speech processes, and in the retention in memory of systems of speech associations. In contrast he found unimpaired the abstract ability to recognize visuospatial or logical relationships.

Hécaen [1962] mentioned disorders of speech typical of left temporal injuries and the difficulty of obtaining solid data for right-sided lesions.

Milner [1958, 1962], with excision studies, found in the left temporal lobe deficits in immediate and delayed recall of verbal material primarily auditory. The right temporal lobe instead showed impairment of retention of nonverbal visual material.

Lansdell [1968], in a factor analysis study of the Wechsler-Bellevue Intelligence Scale in temporal lobe patients, found that the verbal comprehension factor correlated with the extent of left temporal lobe removal but failed to distinguish the side of operation. In addition, a comparison of the 4 most verbal subtest scores (Information, Comprehension, Similarities and Vocabulary) with the other 7 subtests differentiated the side of the lesion within a given sex, indicating a basic difference in the distribution of function between the two sexes.

Dennerll [1964], working with lateralized psychomotor seizure patients, was able to demonstrate with multiple regression scores of Wechsler scales that left-hemisphere subjects showed differential cognitive deficits more clearly than right-hemisphere subjects.

Finally, *Bingley* [1958], in his extensive run of temporal lobe epilepsies and temporal lobe gliomas, concluded that in terms of intellectual impairment in these patients, dominant lobe functions are not limited to the verbal intellectual area because significant impairment in the performance of nonverbal intellectual tasks was observed.

In conclusion, the available findings do not furnish a clear picture of lateralization of functions for many possible reasons among which are: (1) verbal functions of the temporal lobe are primarily represented on the left side, but they are also mediated by the right side; (2) representation of functions in the temporal areas are so plastic that especially between sexes mean studies obscure the findings, and (3) the present understanding of the different components of verbal and intellectual functions in general is totally inadequate to develop outside criteria against which to measure alleged deficits. The present approach therefore is to attempt to analyze the data of this study with a minimum of bias furnished by the previous experiments.

The ubiquity of the 13-Hz activity (except for Picture Completion, Picture Arrangement and Coding) seems to point to a very general component of the functions involved which is not visual and is primarily bilateral in nature. The fact that among the remaining performance subtests the correlations in the temporal areas are higher on the left side, and the verbal subtests (except Comprehension) are higher on the right, could be discounted because of the small differences involved.

Turning to the analysis of the Digit Span and Picture Arrangement subtests, there are some similarities worth noting. For Digit Span (table 9/VI) significant correlations in the 19- and 23-Hz bands were observed in the frontal poles also on the right side. While the more anterior correlations were regarded as relating to the delayed response component of the task, those in the temporal areas could very well be related to a different aspect of short-term memory. *Penfield* [1954] with his stimulation technique had established for the temporal lobe a definite function in memory.

The 15- and 19-Hz significant correlations in the right temporal for Digit Span are also present in the Picture Arrangement subtest with an obvious organizing memory component. Arithmetic shows a primarily left lateralization from 12 to 18 Hz in line with functions described by *Luria* [1966] above.

In regard to the lateralization in the temporal region of the 4 most verbal subtests (Information, Comprehension, Similarities and Vocabulary), the findings are somewhat similar with significance basically from 0 to 14 Hz. Correlations are higher on the right side except for Comprehension in which they are slightly higher on the left. The reason for this latter finding is not clear at present, and the differences are small but consistent throughout the 8 conditions. It should caution researchers about the validity of averaging the scores of the 4 most verbal subtests under the assumption that they are mediated by the same temporal lobe. See chapters 12 and 16 for additional discussion of the functional role of these areas.

Post-Temporal Areas

The placement of these electrodes corresponds to T_3 and T_4 of the 10–20 system. They are located halfway between T_3-O_1 and T_4-O_2, respectively, on the coronal plane. The low significant correlations found in the Full-Scale IQ matrix in the 11- and 13-Hz bands are primarily due to the Verbal IQ components since Performance IQ is noncontributory for these areas. In the Verbal IQ matrix (table 9/XII) significance is found on the right side in the slow bands (1, 3 Hz) and in the alpha band from 8 to 14 Hz. This right-sided preference for verbal material is found in Information and Vocabulary, perhaps reflecting the memory component of these subtests, while Comprehension shows significance in approximately the same frequency with primarily a left-sided preference.

Two other so-called verbal subtests show different patterns. Digit Span (table 9/VI), with a right-lateralization, shows significance in the 1- and 3-Hz bands as for Information, none in the alpha region. The 19-Hz band is also significant for Digit Span in this area as well as in other right brain areas. Arithmetic instead (table 9/III) shows left-sided significance in the 13-, 17-, and 23-Hz bands which also recur in the other brain areas for this subtest. While the lateralization pattern for the 13- and 17-Hz bands is complex, the activity of the 23-Hz band is clearly left-lateralized in all brain areas measured.

The only 2 performance subtests showing significance in these brain areas are Picture Arrangement and Block Design. Picture Arrangement shows limited involvement in the 13- and 17-Hz bands, while Block Design shows the involvement of several bands from 3 to 17 Hz with a clear left lateralization.

In regard to the observed lateralization of the various functions, the stronger left correlations for Arithmetic were expected from observations of deficits consequent to lesions in this area. *Hécaen* [1962] and *Luria* [1966] as well as others found primary arithmetic disturbances or acalculia with lesions of the inferoparietal region. One might readily accept the left lateralization of Comprehension because of its verbal loading, or of Block Design because of its similarity with verbal subtests, but would not have predicted the right lateralization of Information and Vocabulary. Since these 2 latter subtests share similar right-sided significant correlations with Digit Span, the search for a commonality of these 3 subtests would lead to the inference that this brain area on the right side is somehow involved in the retention search or output of information as distinguished from the functions involved in Comprehension and Block Design in which the primary task is more conceptual in nature. So little work has been done in studying these areas that further interpretation of these findings awaits confirmation.

Parietal Areas

The parietal placements (PL, PR) were obtained by trisecting the distance between T_5 and T_6 on a frontal plane. In reference to the 10–20 system, PL is between P_z and P_3 near P_3, while PR is between P_z and P_4 near P_4.

The Full-Scale IQ matrix (table 9/XIV) shows bilateral involvement of 11- and 13-Hz activity and left-sided involvement of higher activity. Performance IQ is noncontributory except for the presence of an isolated left-lateral correlation in the 23-Hz band, while the Verbal IQ pattern is bilateral in the slow (1, 3 Hz) and alpha (11, 13 Hz) bands. These brain areas show the most varied involvement on the part of several subtests. The apparent lack of contribution of the performance subtests is supported by Object Assembly and Coding with no significant correlation but contradicted by Picture Completion with 2 correlations in the 13-Hz band, by Picture Arrangement with correlations from 14 to 20 Hz, and by Block Design with the largest number of correlations in any areas for this subtest. It may therefore be considered a primary area for the performance of this latter task with a primarily left lateralization.

Among the verbal subtests, Digit Span contributes the least with significant correlations in the 1-Hz band, but this finding must have some significance because these 1-Hz correlations are present for the parietal areas in all other verbal subtests (except Arithmetic) as well as Block Design.

While Arithmetic (table 9/III) continues the pattern of demonstrating significant correlations in a fast frequency range (13, 17, and 23 Hz), the remaining 4 most verbal subtests restrict their significance to a low frequency range (0–14 Hz) with Similarities being a poor contributor.

The lateralization pattern of the verbal subtests is primarily bilateral, and it is bilateral for the performance subtests as well except for Block Design where a left-preference is observed especially in the fast frequencies.

The diversity of the patterns of significance obtained is perhaps a consequence of the multiple functions of these areas. *Luria* [1966] quoted *Sechenov* [1891] as originally describing the intellectual disturbances consequent to lesions of the parieto-occipital division of the cortex as pertaining to 'synthesis of individual elements into simultaneous groups'. *Luria* [1966] continued by outlining the scope of these disturbances in visual perception, spatial orientation, logical grammatical operations and calculations which he deemed are closely associated with 'complex forms of spatial analysis and synthesis'.

Luria [1966], *Zeigarnik* [1961], and *Kok* [1960], as well, emphasized the fact that these patients do not lose their symbolic functions or their capacity for abstraction characteristic of frontal lobe injuries but have difficulties consequent to a defect in logical-grammatical operations.

Luria [1966] furthermore focused on the difficulties that these patients have in analyzing spatial relationships and in assembling individual elements into an integrated whole such as in Koh's Block Design test. It should be repeated here that the largest number of significant correlations in Block Design for this study occurs in the parietal areas.

In conclusion, while the presence of deficits consequent to spatial organization on the right side and to aphasia and agraphia on the left side are to be expected, one must not leave this subject without mentioning *Critchley's* [1953] demonstration of the richness and variety of deficits which follow parietal lobe damage and *Arrigoni and De Renzi's* [1964] findings that, when matching for size of parietal lesion, apparent differences between hemispheres disappear, leaving, for example, bilateral deficits in constructional apraxia.

Occipital Poles

The last 2 areas studied which remain to be discussed are the occipital poles. The occipital placements (O_1, O_2 of the 10–20 system) are 1 inch above the inion and, laterally, approximately 1.5 inches from the midline.

The significant correlations obtained with the present method indicate a limited degree of relationship between Full-Scale IQ and EEG power, an isolated 3-Hz correlation on the right side for Verbal IQ, and the largest cluster found in any brain area for Performance IQ, i.e. a row of left-sided correlations in relatively fast frequencies from 12 to 26 Hz.

The individual verbal subtests show: for Comprehension an isolated negative correlation in the 31-Hz band on the right side which occurs also in the adjacent anterior placement in the right post-temporal area, for Vocabulary an isolated right-sided correlation in the 3-Hz band also repeated in several more anterior areas, and for Digit Span similar correlations in the 1- and 3-Hz bands also present in more anterior areas primarily on the right side. Arithmetic shows a different pattern, significant correlations in the 17-, 23-, and 25-Hz bands practically bilateral in nature.

All performance subtests show left-sided preference, albeit with very different patterns. Block Design (table 9/IX) shows the strongest involvement for this area of any of the subtests with 3 clusters of correlations: 1 in the 3-Hz band, 1 in the midrange from 10 to 18 Hz and 1 from 22 to 26 Hz. These correlations and the resulting clusters are almost as strong as the one found for Block Design in the adjacent left post-temporal area.

Picture Arrangement (table 9/VIII) also shows considerable involvement in a frequency range from 12 to 24 Hz. The occipital areas and especially the left occipital represent for Picture Arrangement the area with the largest number of significant correlations, suggesting a primary function of these areas for their conceptual-visual task.

Coding also has in the left occipital area the largest and really the only cluster for this subtest. Significance occurs in the 7-, 17-, 19-, and 23-Hz bands. Picture Completion shows left-sided significance in the 1- and 13-Hz bands, previously observed in other areas for this subtest, as well as in the 17-Hz band, while the only significance for Object Assembly is in the 23-Hz band, which would not be mentioned except for the fact that, for the occipital areas, the correlations of the 23-Hz band reach significance in all the performance subtests.

The correlations obtained indicate that at least in the frequency range studied the occipital poles have an asymmetrical left-preferent role which is primarily restricted to the performance subtests. *De Renzi and Spinnler* [1967] discriminated between perceptual disorders due to language deficits as being consequent to lesions of the left occiput, while similar disorders due to perceptual disorganization occur consequent to right occiput lesions. In this context the frequencies studied would seem to be primarily concerned with the visual-semantic aspects of the performance subtests as well as Arithmetic.

Kinsbourne and Warrington [1963] spoke of simultanagnosia or the deficit of interpreting different features of pictures simultaneously as occurring primarily in left occipital or parieto-occipital regions, a deficit already discussed in the lateral preoccipital section. The correlations obtained in these regions for both Picture Arrangements and Block Design could be related to this function.

Luria [1966] in discussing the intellectual deficits in these areas emphasized that the losses are not of reasoning ability but failed to differentiate clearly between occipital and parieto-occipital areas except for mentioning a paucity of studies of intellectual deficits accompanying optic agnosia.

To conclude this chapter it can be stated that the technique of correlating EEG power and intelligence test subtests has been demonstrated to be of value in attempting to localize and separate components of functions attributed to higher cortical processes. Spectral analysis furnishes a dimensionality that can be used to discriminate and clarify conceptually these different features. This is not the last word on this subject, it is only the beginning of an era in which higher cortical functions can be studied in man without surgical intervention.

References

Arrigoni, G.; De Renzi, E.: Constructional apraxia and hemispheric locus of lesion. Cortex *1:* 170 (1964).

Bingley, T.: Mental symptoms in temporal lobe epilepsy and temporal lobe gliomas. Acta psychiat. neurol. *33:* suppl. 120 (1958).

Brickner, R.M.: The intellectual functions of the frontal lobes (Macmillan, New York 1936).

Cohen, J.: The factorial structure of the WAIS between early adulthood and old age. J. consult. Psychol. *21:* 283–290 (1957a).

Cohen, J.: A factor-analytically based rationale for the Wechsler Adult Intelligence Scale. J. consult. Psychol. *21:* 451–457 (1957b).

Critchley, M.: The parietal lobes (Arnold, London 1953).

Dennerll, R.D.: Prediction of unilateral brain dysfunction using Wechsler test scores. J. consult. Psychol. *28:* 278–284 (1964).

Denny-Brown, D.: The frontal lobes and their functions; in Feeling, Modern trends in neurology (Butterworth, London 1951).

De Renzi, E.; Spinnler, H.: Impaired performance on color tasks in patients with hemispheric damage. Cortex *3:* 194 (1967).

Freeman, W.; Watts, J.W.: Psychosurgery (Thomas, Springfield 1942).

Goldstein, K.: The significance of the frontal lobes for mental performance. J. nerv. Psychopath. *17:* 27–40 (1936).

Hécaen, H.: Clinical symptomatology in right and left hemispheric lesions; in Mountcastle, Interhemispheric relations and cerebral dominance, pp. 215–243 (Johns Hopkins Press, Baltimore 1962).

Kinsbourne, M.; Warrington, E.K.: The localizing significance of limited simultaneous form perception. Brain *86:* 696–702 (1963).

Kok, E.P.: Disturbance of abstraction and spatial direction in the syndrome of the inferior parietal lesion of the dominant hemisphere. Dokl. Akad. Ped. Nauk RSFSR No. 2 (1960).

Landsdell, H.: The use of factor scores from the Wechsler-Bellevue Scale of Intelligence in assessing patients with temporal lobe removals. Cortex *4:* 257–268 (1968).

Luria, A.R.: Higher cortical functions in man (Basic Books, New York 1966).

Luria, A.R.: Frontal lobe syndromes; in Vinken, Bruyn, Handbook of clinical neurology, vol. 2 (Am. Elsevier, New York 1969).

Malmo, R.B.: Interference factors in delayed response in monkeys after removal of frontal lobes. J. Neurophysiol. *5:* 295–308 (1942).

Malmo, R.B.: Psychological aspects of frontal gyrectomy and frontal lobotomy in mental patients. Res. Publs Ass. Res. nerv. ment. Dis. *27:* 537–564 (1948).

Milner, B.: Psychological defects produced by temporal-lobe excision. Res. Publs Ass. Res. nerv. ment. Dis. *36:* 244–257 (1958).

Milner, B.: Laterality effects in audition; in Mountcastle, Interhemispheric relations and cerebral dominance, pp. 177–195 (Johns Hopkins Press, Baltimore 1962).

Penfield, W.: Studies of the cerebral cortex of man. A review and an interpretation; in Delafresnaye, Brain mechanisms and consciousness (Thomas, Springfield 1954).

Pribram, K.: On the neurology of thinking. Behav. Sci. *4:* 265–287 (1959).

Sechenov, I.M.: Physiology of the nervous centers (1891); 2nd ed. (Izd. Akad. Med. Nauk SSSR, Moscow 1952).

Stamm, J.S.; Rosen, S.C.: The locus and crucial time of implication of prefrontal cortex in the delayed response task; in Pribram, Luria, Psychophysiology of the frontal lobes (Academic Press, New York 1973).

Walter, W.G.: The twenty-fourth Maudsley lecture: the functions of the electrical rhythms in the brain. J. ment. Sci. *96:* 1–31 (1950).

Walter, W.G.: The living brain (Norton, New York 1953).

Zeigarnik, B.V.: The pathology of thinking. English translation: Consultants Bureau, New York 1965 (Moscow University Press, Moscow 1961).

12 Factor Analyses of the Wechsler Tests

'... And the worst problem of all was that after a while it was clear neither who was the true "factorman" nor how one could even devise a way of telling who this individual was.'
R.J. Sternberg

In the previous chapter the distribution of patterns of EEG activity relating to intellectual subtests was discussed. A well-known shortcoming of intellectual subtests, however, is the fact that these behavioral scores do not necessarily represent a unitary function, comprised as they are of several components of cognition and perception necessary for executing that function. Coding alone seemed to represent, EEG-wise, a unitary function with activity observed in the left occipital area. It would be highly desirable to be able to separate the several functions into their components and determine their physiological correlates.

To accomplish this, factors obtained from 6 factor-analysis studies of the Wechsler subtests were utilized. With this method it was possible to (1) compare the different factor-analysis studies of the Wechsler tests, and (2) determine the correlates of these factors with EEG parameters.

The method then was to correlate each point in the EEG matrix of values (the EEG matrix consisting of 16 frequency bands for each of 16 brain areas) against factors derived from 6 existing factor-analysis studies of Wechsler tests. Basically these studies (table 10/I) can be divided into 3 groups: (1) a group of 3 studies [*Gault*, 1954; *Cohen*, 1959; *Silverstein*, 1969] based upon the Wechsler Intelligence Scale for Children (WISC) original standardization sample of *Wechsler;* (2) one study of *Davis* [1956] based upon the Wechsler-Bellevue (W-B) test, and (3) a group of 2 studies by *Mundy-Castle* [1958] and *Saunders* [1960] using a South African sample and the African version of the W-B Intelligence Test. The factors developed by *Hammer* [1950] were not included because of their great similarity with the factors developed by *Gault*. Since *Gault* used the WISC and *Hammer* the W-B, *Gault's* study was presumed to be more comparable with the data of the present study.

A summary of the studies' parameters is shown in table 12/I. A total of 32 factors was studied. In addition to the Wechsler scales, some of the studies included other variables in the factor analysis. It was not possible therefore to include the loadings for those variables in the factor scores of our sample. The loadings of significant magnitude were the only ones used to obtain the factor scores for our sample. Only *Mundy-Castle* used also Verbal, Performance and Full-Scale IQ scores in his loadings, and they were used in this study whenever applicable. Also, in Silverstein factor II (table 12/IV) all significant loadings were negative. Therefore, for comparability with other factors of this study, all of the signs of the loadings for that factor were changed to positive.

The significant factor loadings for each of the 32 factors were recorded (tables 12/II–12/V), and factor scores were obtained for each of the subjects in the present study. Correlations were then performed between the EEG power scores and each of the factors in question. The technique is basically the same as the one used for the correlations of EEG power with WISC subtests except that factor scores are substituted for WISC subtests.

By developing factor scores for our subjects and correlating them with each point in the EEG data matrix, it was possible not only to evaluate the physiological structure of each factor for each study but also to compare studies as well and evaluate what these factors relate to in the physiological activity of the brain. The patterns of significant coefficients obtained were very revealing. The factors were grouped into 6 types according to their EEG characteristics as follows:

Type I (table 12/II) resulted in being a ubiquitous pattern characterized by a positive relationship between factor scores and: (1) EEG values somewhere around the 11- to 15-Hz activity and sometimes as low as 9 but primarily 13; (2) a cluster of significant correlations in prefrontal areas in the 19- to 23-Hz frequency bands; (3) a cluster of significant correlations in the frontal areas bilaterally, and (4) a cluster of positive correlations in the 1- to 3-Hz band. Coefficients were primarily stronger on the left side of the homologous pair (e.g. table 12/VI). Type II (table 12/III) is characterized, in addition to strong 11- and 13-Hz activity, by relationships in the 13- to 17-Hz bands in several brain areas (table 12/X). The type III pattern (table 12/IV) is characterized by significant coefficients with EEG power in the 13-Hz band in most brain areas and significant coefficients in the occipital areas in several frequency bands (e.g. table 12/XI). Type IV is characterized

Table 12/I. Factor analysis studies of Wechsler intelligence tests. Factor scores were correlated with EEG power scores in this study. Types refer to patterns of significant coefficients obtained between factor scores and EEG power scores of this study

Author	Test	Age, years–months X̄	Age, years–months range	n	Matrix used	Other tests	Number of factors	I	II	III	IV	V	VI
Gault [1954]	WISC	13–6	13–4 13–8	200	rotated centroid	no	4	1	1	2			
Cohen [1955]	WISC	13–6	13–4 13–8	200	oblique primary	no	5	2	1	2			
Silverstein [1969]	WISC	10–6	7–4 13–8	600	maxplane rotation	no	2	1		1			
Davis [1956]	W-B	12	12–5 16–10	202	orthogonal rotation	yes	10	3	2	5			
Mundy-Castle [1958]	W-B	24		34	rotated centroid	yes	5	3		1	1	1	
Saunders [1960]	W-B	24		34	orthogonal rotation	yes	6	2	2	2			1

Table 12/II. Type I factors and their composition listed in order of increasing significant coefficients in the higher frequency bands

	Type I											Type Ia
	Saunders I Experience	Davis A Verbal comprehension I	Cohen A Verbal comprehension	Mundy-Castle C Age	Gault III Verbal comprehension	Davis K Information	Silverstein I Verbal	Davis E Similarities	Cohen D Verbal comprehension II	Mundy-Castle D Temperamental component	Mundy-Castle B Verbal-abstract	Saunders III Uninterpreted
Information	90	0.42	39	82	51	0.56	67					
Comprehension	44		37	60	48		57		20			
Arithmetic		0.31	26		36	0.32	57		24	40	62	
Similarities					48		60	0.47				
Vocabulary	47	0.60	47	61	51		65					43
Digit Span							41		27	57	40	34
Pict. Compl.												
Pict. Arrang.							31					
Block Design						0.30						
Obj. Ass.												
Coding				42			27				49	57
Verbal IQ							59			62	76	
Perf. IQ												
Full-Scale IQ										64	58	

Table 12/III. Type II factors and their composition listed in order of increasing significant coefficients with EEG scores in the higher frequency bands (11–19 Hz)

	Gault I General eductive	Davis D Mechanical knowledge	Cohen C Freedom from distractibility	Davis F General reasoning
Information	69			
Comprehension	54			
Arithmetic	53	0.34	36	0.33
Similarities	66			0.57
Vocabulary	66			
Digit Span	39	0.34	33	
Pict. Compl.	49			
Pict. Arrang.	51			
Block Design	60	0.41		
Obj. Ass.	49			
Coding	43			
Verbal IQ				
Perf. IQ				
Full-Scale IQ				

by significance in the 5- to 9-Hz activity, stronger on the right side (tables 12/V and 12/XIV). Type V is characterized by a column of negative coefficients in the 9-Hz band (tables 12/V and 12/XV). Type VI is characterized by 6 low-level scattered coefficients (4 of which are negative) with no apparent pattern (tables 12/V, 12/XVI).

Type I Factors

Basically, 12 factors were obtained of this type (cf. table 12/II), the differences being that the first 7 factors had a strong 9-Hz component (even though 11- and 13-Hz coefficients were higher), e.g. *Mundy-Castle's* factor C (table 12/VI) and *Silverstein's* factor I (table 12/VII).

Table 12/VI shows the distribution of significant correlations that occur between the power scores obtained from 64 s of EEG and *Mundy-Castle's* factor C which is primarily loaded on Information, Comprehension and Vocabulary. The pattern reveals correlations in the 9-, 11-, and 13-Hz bands in all but occipital areas and in the 23-Hz band in anterior areas.

The next 2 factors had almost no 9-Hz activity (*Cohen's* factor D, table 12/VIII), and the remaining 2 factors had components from 11 to 15 Hz in addition to the 23-Hz components mentioned above (*Mundy-Castle's* factor B, table 12/IX). The main attributes of type I distribution are primarily

Table 12/IV. Type III factors. Notice the emphasis on numerical and performance subtests and that all 6 studies have a factor with loadings on Picture Completion, Block Design and Object Assembly

	Type III							Type IIIa		Type IIIb		Type IIIc	
	Cohen B Perceptual organization	Mundy-Castle A Practical IQ	Silverstein II Performance	Davis H Perceptual speed	Gault II Spatial-perceptual	Davis B Visualization	Saunders II Deterioration	Davis G Fluency	Gault IV Memory	Davis J Education of conceptual relations	Cohen E Uninterpreted	Saunders VI Uninterpreted	Davis C Numerical facility
Information													
Comprehension													
Arithmetic							+38		30				0.36
Similarities													
Vocabulary								0.37				−58	
Digit Span							+59						
Pict. Compl.	50	64	33		49	0.38						54	
Pict. Arrang.			27		33						33		
Block Design	46	64	53	0.38	56	0.44	+57		38	0.49		64	
Obj. Ass.	57	52	62	0.42	55	0.34						55	
Coding				0.37			+74	0.30			25		0.52
Verbal IQ			40										
Perf. IQ		101											
Full-Scale IQ		68											

Table 12/V. Type IV, V and VI factors (see text)

	Type IV	Type V	Type VI
	Saunders V Uninterpreted	Mundy-Castle E Uninterpreted	Saunders IV Conditioned attention
Information		−30	
Comprehension	−52		
Arithmetic			
Similarities			−42
Vocabulary			
Digit Span			
Pict. Compl.			
Pict. Arrang.	68		42
Block Design		−39	41
Obj. Ass.		48	
Coding		−47	
Verbal IQ			
Perf. IQ			
Full-Scale IQ			

verbal loading and the presence of Arithmetic in those factors in which the higher frequency components are involved. It shows a pattern more weakly observed in the Similarities among the WISC subtests (table 9/IV).

Table 12/I indicates that type I factors are present in most studies, at least once and up to 3 times. Table 12/II shows that these factors were given a broad range of names but primarily were referred to as verbal factors because of their loadings. *Mundy-Castle's* [1958] and *Saunders'* [1960] interpretations of their factors are of interest here because in their studies they used, in addition to W-B subtests, scores of alpha frequency and alpha index. *Mundy-Castle* [1958] obtained 3 type I factors, 1 of which (factor D) is heavily loaded (r = 0.50) on alpha frequency. This finding is mentioned here only anecdotally because the present study does not deal with the distribution of dominant alpha frequency, and comparison with the Mundy-Castle data, on this basis, cannot be made. The fact, however, that all of these 3 factors, B, C and D, produce an almost identical pattern of coefficients with EEG power speaks to the commonality of these factors.

Mundy-Castle [1958] interpreted his factor C as a function of an age component in intelligence. He is erroneous in this because the age factor had been successfully removed by the weighting of the subtest scores, and this weighting was adequate as demonstrated in our study by the age pattern of coefficients (cf. table 8/I). Correlations there are all negative, i.e. orthogonal to the correlations with intellectual subtests which are all positive.

Table 12/VI. *Mundy-Castle's* factor C vs EEG power; significant rhos. This is the first of *Mundy-Castle's* 3 type I factors

		Frequency bands															
		1	3	5	7	9	11	13	15	17	19	21	23	25	27	29	31
Prefrontal	left						·	·					●	·			
	right						·	·					·		·		
Lat. frontal	left						●	●					·				
	right						●	·									
Frontal	left			·		·	●	●	·		·	●	●				
	right	·		●		●	●	●	·	·		·	●	·			
Central	left	●	·			·	●	■									
	right	●				·	●	■									
Temporal	left	·					●	●								−·	
	right	·	·			●	●	●									
Post-temporal	left						·	·									
	right	·	·			·	·										
Parietal	left	·	·				·	·									
	right	·	·				●	●									
Occipital	left																
	right		·														

• Rho with p < 0.05 (0.26–0.34); ● rho with p < 0.01 (0.35–0.42); ● rho with p < 0.001 (0.43–0.48); ■ rho with p < 0.0001 (> 0.48). A minus (–) preceding the dot indicates a negative rho.

Table 12/VII. *Silverstein's* factor I vs EEG power; significant rhos. A type I factor; notice the striking similarity with table 12/VI even though the loadings of these 2 factors are quite different (see table 12/II)

		Frequency bands															
		1	3	5	7	9	11	13	15	17	19	21	23	25	27	29	31
Prefrontal	left						·	·					·	·			
	right						·	·					·		·		
Lat. frontal	left						●	●					·				
	right						●	·	·								
Frontal	left			·		·	●	●	·		·	●	●				
	right	·		●		●	●	●	·	·		·	●				
Central	left	●	·			·	●	■					·				
	right	●					●	■									
Temporal	left						●	●									
	right		·			·	●	■									
Post-temporal	left							·									
	right	·	·			·	·										
Parietal	left	·	·				·	·									
	right	·	·				●	●									
Occipital	left																
	right		·														

• Rho with p < 0.05 (0.26–0.34); ● rho with p < 0.01 (0.35–0.42); ● rho with p < 0.001 (0.43–0.48); ■ rho with p < 0.0001 (> 0.48). A minus (–) preceding the dot indicates a negative rho.

Table 12/VIII. *Cohen's* factor D vs EEG power; significant rhos. One of *Cohen's* type I factors, notice the similarity with tables 12/VI and 12/VII and the difference in the loadings in table 12/II

		Frequency bands															
		1	3	5	7	9	11	13	15	17	19	21	23	25	27	29	31
Prefrontal	left												●	●	•		•
	right												•		•		
Lat. frontal	left						•	●					•				
	right	•											•				
Frontal	left			•				●					•	●			
	right	●		●		•	•	●		•			•				
Central	left	●	•				•	■									
	right	●					•	■						•			
Temporal	left	●					•	●									
	right	●	•				•	●									
Post-temporal	left							•									
	right	•															
Parietal	left		•				•	●		•							
	right	•	•				•	●									
Occipital	left	•															
	right																

• Rho with p < 0.05 (0.26–0.34); ● rho with p < 0.01 (0.35–0.42); ● rho with p < 0.001 (0.43–0.48); ■ rho with p < 0.0001 (> 0.48).
A minus (–) preceding the dot indicates a negative rho.

Table 12/IX. *Mundy-Castle's* factor B vs EEG power; significant rhos. Another of *Mundy-Castle's* type I factors, notice the increase in significance in the 15-Hz band due to a proportionately larger role of the Arithmetic subtest

		Frequency bands															
		1	3	5	7	9	11	13	15	17	19	21	23	25	27	29	31
Prefrontal	left						•	•					•	•			
	right												•		•		
Lat. frontal	left						●	■	•				•				
	right						●	●									
Frontal	left			•			●	■	●		•	•	●				
	right			●		•	●	■	●	•		•	•				
Central	left	●	•				●	■	•								
	right	●					●	■	•					•			
Temporal	left	•					●	■									
	right	•				•	●	■	•							–•	
Post-temporal	left						•	•									
	right	•	•				•										
Parietal	left	•	•				●	●		•						–•	
	right	•	•				●	●	•								
Occipital	left						•										
	right		•														

• Rho with p < 0.05 (0.26–0.34); ● rho with p < 0.01 (0.35–0.42); ● rho with p < 0.001 (0.43–0.48); ■ rho with p < 0.0001 (> 0.48).
A minus (–) preceding the dot indicates a negative rho.

Saunders [1960], in his reanalysis of the Mundy-Castle data, found only one type I factor which he describes as very similar to *Mundy-Castle's* factor C. The only difference between the 2 studies is that *Saunders* did not introduce into the factor analyses the 3 Wechsler IQ scores, Verbal, Performance and Full-Scale, a major criticism of *Mundy-Castle's* analysis.

Davis [1956], among his 10 factors, found 3 of type I having some loadings in other intellectual group tests which he had introduced in his studies.

While *Gault* [1954] and *Silverstein* [1969] have only one type I factor each, *Cohen* [1959] has 2 which he interprets as verbal comprehension I and II. The difference between these factors in our study, observable from the EEG correlations with these factors, is that *Silverstein's* factor I (table 12/VII) has much greater contribution of 9-Hz activity than *Cohen's* factor D (table 12/VIII). From the pattern in table 12/II it seems evident that 9-Hz activity correlates more heavily with subtests of old funds of knowledge such as Information and to a lesser degree Vocabulary and Comprehension. While the presence of 15-Hz activity in the last 2 factors, i.e. *Mundy-Castle's* D and B, is definitely attributable to the presence of the numerical subtests of Arithmetic and Digit Span, the type I appearance of the anterior 23-, 25-, and 27-Hz activity is derived from *Mundy-Castle's* loading on Verbal and Full-Scale IQ.

Saunders' factor III, not a true type I factor, is identified as type IA. It is listed here because of strong correlations in the 11- and 13-Hz bands, but it lacks the characteristic anterior fast activity which is present in all other type I factors. This factor is of particular interest because it appears to represent a more unitary function, EEG-wise, and contains negative correlations in the 29-Hz band, a band which table 8/I shows to be the only one having positive correlations with age.

Type II Factors

Type II seems to be generally associated with the presence of loading in the Arithmetic subtest (cf. table 12/III). This pattern is exemplified by *Davis'* factor F (table 12/X).

The type II factor was not as ubiquitous as type I since it was found only by *Gault* [1954], *Cohen* [1959], and twice by *Davis* [1956]. It is definitely a numerical factor with rather symmetrical distribution in brain areas but with a slight left preference. All 3 authors stay away from a directly

Table 12/X. *Davis's* factor F vs EEG power; significant rhos. The second of *Davis's* type II factors, notice the greater significance of 15- and 17-Hz bands

		Frequency bands															
		1	3	5	7	9	11	13	15	17	19	21	23	25	27	29	31
Prefrontal	left																
	right							•									
Lat. frontal	left				•		●	■	•				●				
	right						•	●	•								
Frontal	left		●	•			•	■	●	•	•	●	●	•			
	right		•			•	•	■	●	●		●	●				
Central	left	●	●				•	■	●	●		•					
	right	•					•	■	●	●				•		•	
Temporal	left	•					●	●	•	•							
	right						•	●	●								
Post-temporal	left			•			•	●	•	●							
	right									●							
Parietal	left		•				•	●	●	●							
	right	•	•				•	●	●	•			•				
Occipital	left																
	right		●														

• Rho with p < 0.05 (0.26–0.34); • rho with p < 0.01 (0.35–0.42); ● rho with p < 0.001 (0.43–0.48); ■ rho with p < 0.0001 (> 0.48). A minus (–) preceding the dot indicates a negative rho.

numerical interpretation of these factors, but from the inspection of the subtest pattern (table 9/III), it seems incontrovertible that the Arithmetic subtest is primarily responsible for the 15- and 17-Hz activity.

A traditional EEG observation is the increase in beta activity (fast EEG activity) during the performance of mental arithmetic. This finding is often attributed to an increase in muscle activity which occurs during the performance of a mental task. The fact that significant beta coefficients were observed with mental arithmetic when correlated with an EEG which was unrelated to the performance of mental Arithmetic (table 9/III) is in support of the hypothesis that increase in beta activity traditionally observed is not necessarily consequent to muscle activity but consequent to mental activity. The interpretation for the current findings would have to be that the general presence of fast activity in the EEG correlates with the possibility for better arithmetic performance when the individual is required to perform such a task.

Type III Factors

Table 12/IV shows that type III factor occurs in the absence of verbal nonnumerical subtests. There are many factors which show this pattern (cf. *Cohen's* factor B, table 12/XI). The variant, type IIIA, is the only one that shows greater significance in the right occipital area rather than the left. Another variant, type IIIB, shows that the significant column of correlations, rather than being in the 13-Hz band, occurs in the 15-, 17- or 19-Hz bands (table 12/XII, e.g. *Cohen's* factor E) and is characterized by the presence of loading in the Picture Arrangement subtest.

A further variant, designated as type IIIC, is characterized by the absence of a column of significance for a given frequency band in several brain areas but retains the presence of significant correlations in the occipital areas, primarily on the left side (cf. table 12/XIII, *Saunders'* factor VI). This latter pattern is similar to that obtained for WISC Coding (table 9/XI).

Table 12/XI. *Cohen's* factor B vs EEG power; significant rhos. A type III factor (see table 12/IV)

		Frequency bands															
		3	5	7	9	11	13	15	17	19	21	23	25	27	29	31	33
Prefrontal	left																
	right																
Lat. frontal	left						•										
	right																
Frontal	left						●										
	right						•										
Central	left						■										
	right						●										
Temporal	left						●										
	right																
Post-temporal	left						•										–•
	right																
Parietal	left						●					●					
	right						●										
Occipital	left					•	●		•			●	•				
	right																

• Rho with p < 0.05 (0.26–0.34); ● rho with p < 0.01 (0.35–0.42); ● rho with p < 0.001 (0.43–0.48); ■ rho with p < 0.0001 (> 0.48). A minus (–) preceding the dot indicates a negative rho.

Table 12/XII. *Cohen's* factor E vs EGG power; significant rhos. A type IIIB factor, a variant of type III

| | | \multicolumn{16}{c}{Frequency bands} | | | | | | | | | | | | | | |
		1	3	5	7	9	11	13	15	17	19	21	23	25	27	29	31
Prefrontal	left																
	right																
Lat. frontal	left		−•	−•													
	right		−•	−●	−•												
Frontal	left		−●														
	right		−•														
Central	left										•						
	right										•						
Temporal	left																
	right																
Post-temporal	left																
	right																
Parietal	left										•						
	right										•						
Occipital	left									●	●	•	●	•			
	right									●	●	•	•	•			

• Rho with p < 0.05 (0.26–0.34); ● rho with p < 0.01 (0.35–0.42); ● rho with p < 0.001 (0.43–0.48); ■ rho with p < 0.0001 (> 0.48).
A minus (−) preceding the dot indicates a negative rho.

Table 12/XIII. *Saunders'* factor VI vs EEG power; significant rhos. A type IIIC factor, it is loaded on the same subtests as *Cohen's* factor B (table 12/XI) but in addition is negatively loaded on Vocabulary. Note that with that change the significant coefficients in the 13-Hz band are removed

| | | \multicolumn{16}{c}{Frequency bands} | | | | | | | | | | | | | | |
		3	5	7	9	11	13	15	17	19	21	23	25	27	29	31	33
Prefrontal	left																
	right																
Lat. frontal	left																
	right																
Frontal	left																
	right																
Central	left						•						•				
	right																
Temporal	left																
	right																
Post-temporal	left																
	right																
Parietal	left											•					−•
	right																
Occipital	left						•		•			●	•				
	right																

• Rho with p < 0.05 (0.26–0.34); ● rho with p < 0.01 (0.35–0.42); ● rho with p < 0.001 (0.43–0.48); ■ rho with p < 0.0001 (> 0.48).
A minus (−) preceding the dot indicates a negative rho.

Among the WISC studies, *Gault* and *Cohen* isolated one type III and one type IIIB factor, the IIIB constituting a factor which includes the 15- to 19-Hz activity (*Cohen's* factor E showing only 19-Hz activity), while *Silverstein* isolated only one type III factor.

What is unique in *Cohen's* factor E (table 12/XII) is the cluster of negative coefficients in frontal and lateral frontal areas. A large portion of EEG power in these areas is attributed to eye-movement artifacts readily discernable in the raw EEG because of their high amplitude. In spectral analysis, eye-muscle potential typically clusters in anterior brain areas in the low frequency bands. Subjects vary in the degree to which eye-movement artifacts increase during the performance of mental arithmetic (as observed earlier, chapter 9) in the Coding subtest (table 9/XI), and the degree of this increase was negatively correlated with successful performance on Coding. *Cohen's* factor E is loaded on both Coding and Picture Arrangements (tables 9/XI and 9/VIII), both showing a vestige of significant negative correlations in the anterior low frequencies.

It could be argued that by combining Picture Arrangement and Coding this negative anterior activity becomes potentiated and points to the interpretation that Picture Arrangement as well as Coding become penalized by the presence of random eye movement. In this experiment, however, the correlations with *Cohen's* factor E as well as with all other factors were with a baseline EEG, not an EEG recorded during the performance of the Coding or Picture Arrangement subtests. Any correlations, therefore, are not a relationship with EEG power consequent to the task in question but indicate the presence in the EEG baseline of an activity which correlates with the capacity for the performance of the intellectual task in question whenever required. Since only 8 s of the 64-second of EEG were recorded during the performance of mental Arithmetic (cf. chapter 9), it seems improbable that negative significance could be reached because of the 8-second mental arithmetic component. It is then necessary that differences in the amount of eye movement in the baseline EEG are sufficient to predict performance in Coding or Picture Arrangement.

Among the intellectual tasks not pertaining to the WISC, this anterior cluster of negative coefficients in low frequency bands was observed only in the Psychomotor task (table 10/IV). In both the Psychomotor task and in Coding the task can be carried out effectively with quick, directed eye movements. If the servomechanism for these eye movements is poor, the subject is penalized by lower speed in the performance of the task. It seems that in Picture Arrangement the same facility is involved in that purposeful eye movements need to be directed effectively to different portions of the figures to isolate the pertinent features. Poor visual tracking reduces the speed of performance in these timed tasks by penalizing the subject who has to process and repeatedly discard the irrelevant features of the drawings in Picture Arrangement or the wrong symbol in the Coding subtest.

Factor E, then, for which *Cohen* did not find a specific meaning, could have been isolated because of its role in presiding over this visuomotor function which correlates negatively with performance on WISC Picture Arrangement, Coding and the Psychomotor task of this study.

Davis, with his 10 factors, has 5 factors of type III, among which only one factor type IIIA is characterized by right occipital involvement. Since, of the 2 loadings of this factor, the Coding subtest shows primarily left occipital involvement (table 9/XI) and Digit Span primarily right involvement (table 9/V), the contribution of the right occipital involvement seems to be primarily due to Digit Span (table 9/VI).

Mundy-Castle's analysis has only 1 type III factor, factor A, which, because it is his first factor, accounts for the greatest amount of variance in his study. This factor has a positive loading on alpha frequency and a negative loading on alpha index (a measure which is related to amplitude of dominant alpha activity). The present study does not deal with the distribution of dominant alpha frequency, but the negative loading of the alpha index does not find support in our data. In as much as alpha index can be regarded as a measure of dominant alpha amplitude, there is no evidence of negative coefficients between 11-Hz activity (dominant alpha in the present study) and the performance subtests which load *Mundy-Castle's* factor A (tables 12/IV, 9/VII, 9/IX, 9/X, 9/XIII and 9/XIV).

Of *Saunders'* 2 type III factors, factor II has similar loadings to *Mundy-Castle's* factor A but obtains a larger number of significant coefficients. *Saunders'* factor VI (table 12/XIII) is classified here as a variant of type III factors (type IIIC) because it retains the left occipital significant correlations of type III factors but not the column of 13-Hz significant correlations. The distribution of correlations of this factor acquires particular relevance when compared with that of *Cohen's* factor B (table 12/XI). They both have positive loadings on Picture Completion, Block Design and Object Assembly, but *Saunders'* factor VI, in addition, is negatively loaded on Vocabulary.

One could easily conclude that introducing a negatively loaded Vocabulary to the 3 subtests of *Cohen's* factor B is equivalent to removing the verbal component from those 3 performance subtests. The observed EEG result is the removal of the significance of the 13-Hz frequency band throughout brain areas. It should be emphasized at this point that these 2 tables are not a result of manipulations of the loadings performed by the present investigator, but they are the EEG correlates of factors which were found in the factor analysis of the Wechsler tests performed by *Saunders* and *Cohen,* respectively.

The distribution of significant correlations of the type III factors leads to questioning whether these factors are representative of a unitary function. Significant occipital activity as originating from visual projection areas could have been predicted for visual functions such as Picture Completion, Block Design and Object Assembly. What is surprising is the clustering of the significant correlations in the left of the 2 occipital areas. This finding clearly points to a dominant role of the left occipital area for this activity. Differential reliability between the EEGs from the left and right occipital areas does not seem to play a role here (table 3/III).

The question arose as to whether 13-Hz activity constituted a correlate of the intellectual *'g'* factor, ubiquitous in intelligence scores. All that can be concluded here is that the negative loading of Vocabulary in *Saunders'* factor VI is tantamount to subtracting the verbal component from *Cohen's* factor B. The removal of the significance of the 13-Hz activity in *Saunders'* factor VI clearly demonstrates a functional role of the 13-Hz activity for verbal processing.

Incidence of Type IV, V and VI Factors

In addition to the first 3 factor types, *Saunders'* factor V is the only type IV factor. It is the only factor characterized by significance in the 5- to 9-Hz activity, stronger on the right side and positively loaded on Picture Arrangement and negatively loaded on Comprehension (table 12/XIV).

Another unique factor is represented as type V by *Mundy-Castle's* factor E (table 12/XV). It shows a column of negative correlations in the 9-Hz band related to the relationship between positive loading on Object Assembly and negative loading on Information, Picture Arrangement and Coding.

Last is *Saunders'* factor IV, referred to as type VI, which has a total of 6 low-level scattered correlations, 4 of which are negative with no apparent pattern (table 12/XVI).

It is relevant to note that the findings discussed so far are based on identical sets of EEG data correlated with either subtest scores or factor scores. This EEG data was obtained under a set of conditions unrelated to

Table 12/XIV. *Saunders'* factor V vs EEG power; significant rhos. The type IV factor (see table 12/V)

		Frequency bands															
		1	3	5	7	9	11	13	15	17	19	21	23	25	27	29	31
Prefrontal	left																
	right				•								•				
Lat. frontal	left			•	●			•					•				
	right			•	●												
Frontal	left			•	●	•		•					•				
	right			•	●	●		•					●	•			
Central	left	•	•	•	•	•											
	right			•	•	•											
Temporal	left	•		●	●	•											
	right			●	●												
Post-temporal	left			•	●												
	right			•	•												−•
Parietal	left			•	•												
	right		•	•	•	•											−•
Occipital	left										−•						
	right																−●

• Rho with p < 0.05 (0.26–0.34); ● rho with p < 0.01 (0.35–0.42); ● rho with p < 0.001 (0.43–0.48); ■ rho with p < 0.0001 (> 0.48).
A minus (–) preceding the dot indicates a negative rho.

Table 12/XV. *Mundy-Castle's* factor E vs EEG power; significant rhos. The type V factor (see table 12/V)

		Frequency bands															
		1	3	5	7	9	11	13	15	17	19	21	23	25	27	29	31
Prefrontal	left		•														
	right																
Lat. frontal	left		●														
	right		•	•		−•											
Frontal	left		•			−•											
	right					−•					−•						
Central	left					−•											
	right					−•											
Temporal	left		•			−•											
	right					−•											
Post-temporal	left					−•											
	right					−•	−•										
Parietal	left					−•											
	right										−•						
Occipital	left					−•				−•							
	right		−•			−•				−•	−•						

• Rho with p < 0.05 (0.26–0.34); ● rho with p < 0.01 (0.35–0.42); ● rho with p < 0.001 (0.43–0.48); ■ rho with p < 0.0001 (> 0.48).
A minus (–) preceding the dot indicates a negative rho.

Table 12/XVI. *Saunders'* factor IV vs EEG power; significant rhos. The type VI factor (see table 12/V)

		\multicolumn{16}{c}{Frequency bands}														
		3	5	7	9	11	13	15	17	19	21	23	25	27	29	31	33
Prefrontal	left																•
	right																
Lat. frontal	left																
	right			−•								−•					
Frontal	left																
	right			−•													•
Central	left																
	right																
Temporal	left																
	right																
Post-temporal	left																
	right																
Parietal	left																
	right		−•														
Occipital	left																
	right																

• Rho with p < 0.05 (0.26–0.34); ● rho with p < 0.01 (0.35–0.42); ● rho with p < 0.001 (0.43–0.48); ■ rho with p < 0.0001 (> 0.48). A minus (–) preceding the dot indicates a negative rho.

the subtests. The correlations obtained therefore are not the resultant of EEG activity consequent to the functions of the variable involved. They comprise components of ongoing EEG activity which constitute the sine qua non for the performance of the correlated function. This research technique was used because it was felt that in this manner, if any correlations could be found, they would have to be due to the capacity for performing the subtest involved and not to some artifactual relationship with other unaccounted variables.

In summary, results showed: (1) patterns of significant correlations indicating a considerable degree of similarity between factors of different studies; (2) 2 or more factors in a given study having nearly identical patterns of significant correlations, indicating that these factors obtained with varying contributions of the different subtests were, at least electrophysiologically, identical, and (3) an indication that each of these factors is not electrophysiologically unitary but is composed of more than 1 cluster of activity organized around a given frequency band or a given brain area.

If one were to work back from the data, i.e. extrapolate EEG factors from the patterns of relationships between EEG parameters and intellectual factors, the following factors could be extracted from a visual inspection of the matrices:

(1) age, resulting in the decrease in all but alpha frequencies with increase in age;

(2) general-verbal, represented by the presence of 13-Hz power;

(3) problem-solving, represented by the presence of 17-Hz power (15- to 19-Hz bands) which correlates with the story problems of Arithmetic and Picture Arrangement;

(4) general II, represented by the presence of 23-Hz power which correlates primarily with anterior brain areas in verbal subtests and posterior brain areas with performance subtests;

(5) performance, represented by the presence of power in primarily left occipital areas in a broad range of frequencies, and

(6) muscular coordination, inferred by eye-movement artifacts in 1- to 5-Hz bands, in anterior brain areas. These EEG artifacts correlate negatively with performance on Coding, Picture Arrangement of the WISC and the psychomotor task.

In light of the overwhelming similarity of EEG patterns derived from diverse compositions of intellectual factors and of the negative correlations between EEG power and age, in conjunction with positive correlations between EEG power and intellectual variables, the issue of intellectual factor changes through life can be studied in a new light. The issue arises from the observation of apparent age-related changes in the factor structure of intelligence. As *Reinert* [1970] points out, the available evidence has led to several hypotheses variously attributing the factor changes to age [*Burt*, 1919; *Garrett*, 1946], ability levels, or ontogenetic variables as a whole [*Spearman*, 1927]. Such hypotheses are in direct contradiction with models relying upon a general invariance of intelligence structure [*Thurstone*, 1938; *Guilford*, 1967].

The patterning of EEG power as related to intellectual factor scores observed in the present study would indicate that some of the factor changes observed in the literature may not be physiologically relevant or may be an artifact of the factor analytic technique even though the presence of 2 identical EEG patterns does not prove that the 2 factors are identical. The inverse relationship between age (table 8/I) and intelligence (tables 9/I–9/XIV), however, can be used to separate age components from other developmental components heretofore considered to be parallel parameters.

In conclusion, the methodology of the present study is suggested as a powerful technique for testing the validity of theoretical assertions that heretofore could only be studied inferentially.

References

Burt, C.: The bearing of the factor theory on the organization of schools and classes. Report of the LCC Psychologist (London 1919).

Cohen, J.: The factorial structure of the WISC at ages 7–6, 10–6, and 13–6. J. consult. Psychol. *23:* 285–299 (1959).

Davis, P.C.: A factor analysis of the Wechsler-Bellevue Scale.. Educ. psychol. Measmt *16:* 127–146 (1956).

Garrett, H.E.: A developmental theory of intelligence. Am. Psychol. *1:* 372–378 (1946).

Gault, U.: Factorial patterns of the Wechsler intelligence scales. Aust. J. Psychol. *6:* 85–89 (1954).

Guilford, J.P.: The nature of human intelligence (McGraw-Hill, New York 1967).

Hammer, A.G.: A factorial analysis of the Bellevue intelligence tests. Aust. J. Psychol. *1:* 108–114 (1950).

Mundy-Castle, A.C.: Electrophysiological correlates of intelligence. J. Personality *26:* 184–199 (1958).

Reinert, G.: Comparative factor analytic studies of intelligence throughout the human life-span; in Goulet, Baltes, Life-span developmental psychology, pp. 467–484 (Academic Press, New York 1970).

Saunders, D.R.: Further implications of Mundy-Castle's correlations between EEG and Wechsler-Bellevue variables. J. natn. Inst. Personnel Res. *8:* 91–101 (1960).

Silverstein, A.B.: An alternative factor analytic solution for Wechsler's intelligence scales. Educ. psychol. Measmt *29:* 763–767 (1969).

Spearman, C.: The abilities of man (Macmillan, London 1927).

Thurstone, L.L.: Primary mental abilities (University of Chicago Press, Chicago 1938).

13 Regional Spectral Analysis of EEG and 'Active' and 'Passive' Intelligence

W.T. Liberson

'Law is order.'
Aristotle

The purpose of this chapter is to integrate some of the information presented in this book by *Giannitrapani* with the related research published by me during the past several decades. A second purpose is to summarize our conjoint effort to analyze the results of his studies in the light of those of my current investigations that seem to contribute to the content of this monograph. All references to the work of *Giannitrapani* made in this chapter concern the information presented by him in this book.

In the late 1930s I observed that correlations of some EEG parameters with the scores earned in various tests of intelligence differ according to the nature of the subtests.

Thus, for example, in normal individuals [railroad engineers; *Liberson, 1941*] those subjects who were characterized by a 'dominant' type of EEG [according to the early classification of *Davis and Davis, 1936*] had significantly better achievement in some tests of technical ability and short memory than subjects characterized by a 'mixed' type of EEG (lesser and more irregular alpha activity). Yet no difference was found between these two types of subjects insofar as other tests of intelligence were concerned, for example, a test of 'general intelligence'.

Later, examining more than 300 mental patients, both neurotic and psychotic, a negative relationship was found between the presence of diffuse EEG abnormality and achievement on the subtest of 'conceptual' ability of *Shipley's* [1940] test, while the scores on vocabulary were not similarly affected. During this study [*Liberson, 1950, 1951, 1967*] it was noted that while the scores of the vocabulary subtest declined only after age 60, an early decline at the age of 40 was found for the subtest of 'conceptual' ability. In considering alpha frequency distribution as a function of age in the same kind of population [*Liberson, 1951, 1967*], a flattening of the distribution above the age of 50 and a bimodality of this distribution above the age of 60 was found. The number of 'movement' responses on the Rorschach test was found to be the only parameter on that test that shows the same kind of decline with age as 'performance' or 'conceptual' test scores.

Since that time, it has become known to clinical psychologists that an index of 'organicity' in mental patients is the discrepancy between performance and verbal scores. The same kind of discrepancy between Performance and Verbal IQ is found with aging.

In 1951 I postulated two types of intelligence tests [*Liberson*, 1951]: those evaluating 'active' intelligence such as performance or conceptual tests and those of 'passive' intelligence, such as vocabulary. It was felt that this dichotomy was more useful than a definition of the Performance and Verbal IQ. The latter includes such subtests as Arithmetic which involves activity that is clearly consistent with 'active' intelligence.

This point was discussed at length in the PhD thesis [*Liberson*, 1950; see also 1951, 1967]: 'the presence of dissociation between "passive" and "active" intelligence (as expressed respectively in scores on vocabulary and conceptual subtests) suggests that the latter requires for its efficiency the participation of processes and structures from which the former is less dependent. The simplest hypothesis is that there are related processes of activation analogous to the physiological tone which is observed at various levels of neurophysiological activity. The finding that a decrease of "active" intelligence is associated with a disturbance of electrical activity in the brain suggests that neural formations which participate in the activation of intelligence are the same, at least in part, as those which interfere with the synchronous electrical activity of the cortex. It is known that the latter is influenced by regulating centers located in the thalamus and hypothalamus. One is led to conclude that the participation of these centers, dynamically related to the cortex and the basal ganglia, are essential for the preservation of "active" intelligence. Until now, the neurological approach to intelligence has been limited to the study of different cortical areas; the participation of diencephalic regions has been left completely in the dark ... These centers could act upon different areas of the cortex according to a predetermined gradient. Thus the importance of different regions of the cortex in the persistence of intellectual efficiency may be partially explained.'

More recently *Liberson* [1967] added that 'in the light of *Magoun's* and *Moruzzi's* investigation [see *Magoun*, 1963], the mesencephalic region should be added to the thalamus and hypothalamus'. One might also add now that some hippocampal structures participate in some cognitive functions.

The following personal experimental observations seem to contribute to this hypothesis:

(1) In collaboration with *Strauss* et al. [1943] we found that, in psychoneurotics presumably subject to emotional turmoil involving deeper regions of the brain, alpha activity is often depressed over the left parieto-occipital region. This first observation of hemispheric differences under stress was further confirmed by me in the following observations: (a) In many cases of mental patients performing the serial 7s test, alpha rhythm in the left parieto-occipital region was more depressed than in the right one. (b) In patients following electric shock treatments, the left parieto-occipital region showed less post-treatment slow activity than the rest of the brain. (c) In some patients showing diffuse 'sleep pattern', the left parietal region showed intermittent alpha activity.

(2) In other observations 'alpha power' was positively correlated with intelligence just as in the first paper on railroad engineers. Thus: (a) In a recent article [*Liberson and Fried*, 1981], we showed that inhabitants of a nursing home who lacked in their parieto-occipital EEG any significant frequency component above 7 Hz were judged by the therapists as intellectually incompetent. (b) In 1937, *Chweitzer* et al. found that mescaline, a hallucinogenic substance that also considerably decreases intellectual abilities, lowers 'alpha power'. In 1936 *Liberson* had introduced the measurement of 'alpha power' by making histograms of amplitudes of alpha waves in the parieto-occipital region. This methodology was also used much more recently by *Goldstein* [1981] who confirmed our findings and refined our methodology. He showed that 'alpha power' in the temporal region, expressed by a histogram similar to ours, showed an increase of multimodality in patients with schizophrenia or depression and therefore a decrease of underlying control although with different left-right hemispheric predominance. (c) In an article [*Liberson and Liberson*, 1966], we reported that as soon as 'alert' alpha rhythm was suspended, mental content of our subjects shifted from concrete to vague.

There was an apparent contradiction in all these findings. On the one hand a higher 'alpha power' seemed to favor performance; on the other hand *during* performance or excitement, certain brain wave areas showed a depression of alpha power. This contradiction could be resolved by assuming at that time that the apparent depression of alpha power is related to the speeding up of brain wave frequencies. Thus, the importance of brain wave

frequencies and of their differential localization in the cortex became paramount.

The material gathered and analyzed by *Giannitrapani* seems to be particularly suited for checking some of my previous hypotheses. If indeed
subcortical 'driving' of the cortex expresses itself in increasing brain wave
frequency, then performance test scores must be positively correlated with
faster rhythms while 'passive' intelligence may exhibit high correlations
with theta or lower or mid-alpha frequency rhythms. If there is a preferential cortical region involved for success in a particular intelligence test, then
the EEG requirement to be fulfilled is to offer at that site adequate brain
wave frequency, relatively slow for 'passive' intelligence and sufficiently
high for 'active' intelligence of a particular type. This is exactly what is
revealed by the analysis of *Giannitrapani's* data. Obviously, one must distinguish a propensity for success in a test of intelligence from actual EEG
changes during its administration.

The tables prepared by *Giannitrapani* portray the strength of the correlations of each test score with brain wave frequency recorded in each particular area of the scalp. In order to simplify the study, I divided the scalp
into three areas: frontal, centrotemporal and posterior (posterior temporal,
parietal and occipital).

Regional Correlative Strength

The size of the dots in the tables of chapter 9 increases with the strength
of the correlations between EEG power and achievement in any given subtest. The size of the dot corresponds to the degree of significance of the
correlations at least at the 0.26 level. It is possible to develop a score by
attributing weight to the significance levels in question. If the smallest dot is
given a weight of 1 and the larger dots weights of 2, 3 and 4, respectively, the
total number obtained in a particular frequency range is therefore a measurement of the corresponding correlative strength. One other method is to
add algebraically all the coefficients of correlations (rhos) for a particular
test and a particular region or hemisphere. Both methods permit one to
define the regional *correlative* strength of a particular brain wave frequency
with a specific subtest.

First, I considered the regional correlative strength of different EEG
frequencies with the following subtests: (1) Vocabulary; (2) Information; (3)
Comprehension; (4) Similarities; (5) Arithmetic; (6) Block Design; (7) Digit

Span; (8) Picture Completion, and (9) Picture Arrangement. The other subtests were not considered here because of the small number of significant correlations.

The last 3 subtests are usually considered as contributing to Performance IQ while the first 6 subtests contribute to Verbal IQ. As mentioned above and discussed in chapters 9 and 16 by *Giannitrapani*, Arithmetic may be considered separately from the other verbal tests, being a test of 'active' intelligence. Moreover, Block Design might also be considered as requiring processes of 'active' intelligence.

Figures 13/1 and 13/2 show that, in general, distributions of various brain wave frequencies' correlative strength are different from what is known on the basis of classical electroencephalography.

Figure 13/1 illustrates 2 major findings: (1) frequency peaks of 'raw' EEG are not the same as those revealed by the study of correlations between intelligence and brain wave frequency; (2) spatial distribution of brain wave activity of different frequency bands are not the same in the 'raw' EEG and in the EEG components that correlate with intelligence.

As far as the frequency is concerned, the raw EEG shows marked peaks of 9–11 and 29 Hz as well as small 'humps' at the 17- and 21-Hz frequency bands. Correlative EEG shows predominantly peaks of 13, 17, and 23 Hz.

As far as the topography is concerned, the raw EEG shows predominance of both slow and beta frequencies in the frontal regions while alpha rhythm (9–11 Hz) predominates in the posterior region. 'Correlative EEG' shows predominance of 13-Hz activity in the centrotemporal region, followed by frontal cortex and, to a lesser degree, the posterior region. In contradistinction to this, 17 Hz predominates in the posterior region, followed by the centrotemporal region. It is absent in the frontal region.

29- and 21-Hz activities are replaced by 23-Hz beta rhythm predominating by far in the frontal region, followed by the centrotemporal region and represented by a small 'hump' in the posterior area of the convexity.

The most impressive findings are the absence of significant correlative strength with intelligence of the slow alpha rhythm, especially in the posterior regions where this rhythm predominates in the 'raw' EEG, and the shift of the correlative strength from the 29- to the 23-Hz beta band. Both keep their frontal predominance while the emerging 17-Hz beta activity is almost restricted to the posterior regions. These findings stress the functional significance of different frequency bands as well as their localization and also the necessity of extracting these 'privileged' frequencies by special correlative techniques so successfully carried out by *Giannitrapani*.

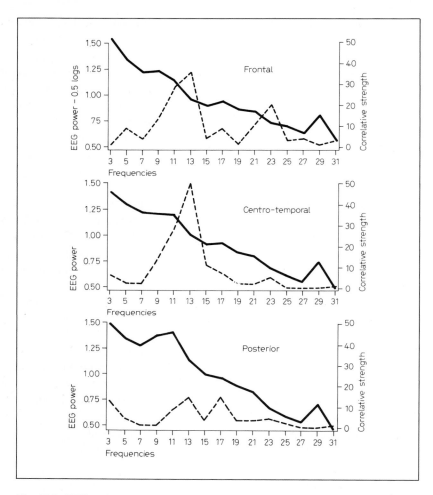

Fig. 13/1. EEG power spectral activity and correlative strength in the frontal, centro-temporal and posterior regions. The power spectrum is expressed in 0.5 log units; the correlative strength in weighted dots derived from the tables in chapter 9. ——— = EEG power; – – – = correlative strength.

Figure 13/2 represents the same findings with more emphasis on 'local signs'. On the left side (raw EEG) beta activity from 23 to 27 Hz is shown predominating over the frontal region. With the advent of 21-Hz activity, going down to 17-Hz rhythm, there is an increasing presence of beta rhythm over the posterior convexity equaling that present over the frontal brain.

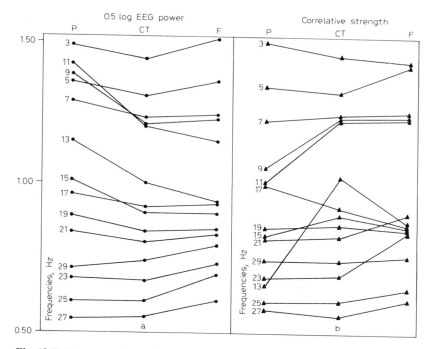

Fig. 13/2. The same data as in figure 13/1. However, they are represented here as spatial profiles for 3 investigated regions. The units of the vertical scale are the same as in figure 1. The level of 'profiles' of the correlative strength of different frequencies is chosen in the following way. For each frequency the level of the correlative strength found for the centrotemporal region in **b** is aligned with the level of the EEG power for the same region represented in **a**. From this point, taken for 0, greater or smaller strengths are counted upward or downward as the case may be for the frontal and posterior regions.

This process of 'posteriorization' of brain wave activity is accentuated in the 15-, 13-, 11-, and 9-Hz rhythms. Then starting with 7-Hz rhythm, this posterior predominance lessens and for 5- and 3-Hz slow activities shows equal presence on both frontal and posterior regions, reaching the minimum over the central region.

This topography is radically changed for the brain wave frequency correlating with intelligence on the right side of figure 13/2. Again going downward, the 21- and particularly the 23-Hz beta rhythm show a selective increase over the frontal convexity. This trend is suddenly interrupted for 19-Hz rhythm and for 17-Hz frequency when a sudden predominance over

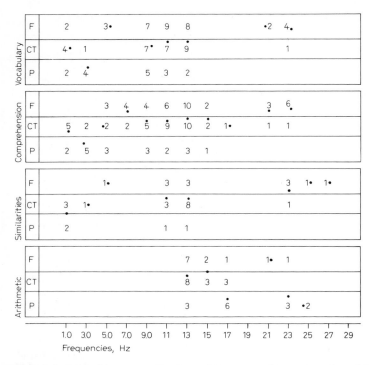

Fig. 13/3a. This figure represents 'correlative strength' as a function of brain wave frequency and region (F = frontal; CT = centrotemporal; P = posterior) for 3 subtests of 'passive' intelligence (Vocabulary, Comprehension and Similarities) and one of 'active' intelligence (Arithmetic) figured here for comparison. Numbers represent the weighted values of the dots in the tables of chapter 9. The dots in this figure represent the weighted location of the correlative strength.

the occipital region emerges. However, just as suddenly, the posterior presence of 9- to 15-Hz rhythms, as a frequency correlating with intelligence, ceases. The frequencies of this order that correlate with intelligence predominate on the central cortex (particularly 13- and 15-Hz frequencies) and then are equally present on the centrotemporal-frontal convexity. While the presence of 5-Hz frequency increases for the frontal cortex, the 3-Hz activity shows its maximum on the occipital and its minimum on the frontal cortex.

All these findings stress the limitation of considering the relationship of 'raw' EEG frequency spectrum to intelligence, a state of affairs that has existed prior to the study of *Giannitrapani*.

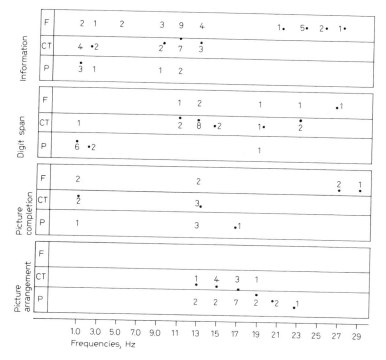

Fig. 13/3b. The same notations as for **a**; however, 3 subtests of 'active' intelligence (Digit Span, Picture Completion and Picture Arrangement) are compared to one test of 'passive' intelligence (Information).

To summarize, the 'correlative strength' of 3-Hz slow waves predominates in the posterior half of the head instead of the usual centrofrontal regions. Alpha correlative strength predominates in the centrotemporal region instead of its usual occipital predominance. Beta correlative strength shows, in addition to the usual frontal predominance, a predilection for the posterior region in cases of 'active' intelligence involving visual functions.

Figure 13/3a, b shows 'correlative strength' as a function of both brain regions and brain wave frequency for tests of 'passive' and 'active' intelligence. In figure 13a, 3 representative subtests of 'passive' intelligence are compared with one representative test of 'active' intelligence (Arithmetic).

Conversely in figure 13/3b, 3 representative tests of 'active' intelligence are compared with one representative of 'passive' intelligence. It can be seen from these figures that: (1) Generally, correlative strength involves more anterior regions as the correlative frequency increases with one notable exception, the test for Picture Arrangement where faster frequencies seem to involve posterior regions, no doubt because of the involved visual function. The same trend is seen partially for Picture Completion and for Arithmetic. The latter finding suggests the importance of visual representation in arithmetic performance. (2) Activity between 3 and 9 Hz is generally absent for tests of 'active' intelligence. In the case of Picture Arrangement and Arithmetic no slow activity correlates with performance in these tests.

Figure 13/4 shows combined correlative strength of brain wave frequency as a function of brain region. The same tendency of progressively higher frequency with advancing forward location is seen in this graph. However, this trend is interrupted by a posterior 'dip' chiefly involving 17-Hz rhythm preferentially present, as stated above, in the posterior regions. However, 13 and 15 Hz are also partially involved in this 'dip'. The movement forward of the correlative strength of faster frequencies is seen again above the level of 17-Hz frequency.

Let us mention that 'passive' intelligence shows a number of negative correlations with beta activity (above 20 Hz).

Alpha-Plus Frequencies

If one considers only brain wave frequencies between 8 and 20 Hz one may feel more secure in avoiding artifacts of noncerebral origin, for example, eye movements for slow frequencies and muscle potentials for the faster ones. This does not imply that the results spelled out by *Giannitrapani* and those discussed above in this chapter are to be mistrusted. There is no way I can explain definitive correlations found, for example, for posterior slow activity with intelligence by mere artifacts.

However, let us consider, as did *Giannitrapani,* the regional correlative strength of each of the 8- to 20-Hz frequency bands for each subtest of the Wechsler Intelligence Scale for Children (WISC). Again I lumped together broader regions of the scalp than those represented by *Giannitrapani* in the tables of chapter 9.

For some of these subtests detailed histograms representing distributions of the correlative strength (ordinates) for each frequency band, as well

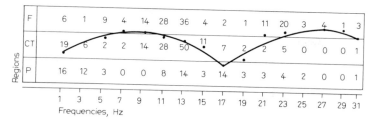

Fig. 13/4. Same notation as for figure 13/3a, b. However, in this figure a combined correlative strength of brain wave frequencies is considered for all tests of intelligence.

as for the 3 regions of the scalp, were obtained separately for the left and right hemispheres (fig. 13/5).

Slower frequencies were found to have greater correlative strength for 'passive' than for 'active' intelligence subtests. The latter show greater correlative strength with the higher frequencies.

Vocabulary. This indeed appears as the most 'passive' intelligence manifestation, more than any other subtest. Note on the histogram for this subtest an abrupt drop in correlative strength in frequencies above 14 Hz in either hemisphere. Average correlative frequency is 12.1 Hz both on the left and right sides. For this figure the 'correlative' strength was calculated by averaging all the coefficients of correlation together no matter how significant they were. This was done separately for the anterior, intermediate (centrotemporal) and posterior regions.

Information. This is another subtest of 'passive' intelligence having a correlative average frequency of 12.4 Hz. The same drop in correlative strength was observed above the frequency of 14 Hz as for Vocabulary.

Comprehension. This test seems to involve a somewhat higher degree of activity. Consequently it correlates with 15-Hz activity in a greater proportion of cases than for the subtests considered above. The average correlated frequency, however, is still relatively low, 12.8 Hz.

Similarities. This subtest appears to require a greater amount of 'driving' than the previous 3 subtests. It depends on more 'activated' brain wave frequencies as the average frequency with which it correlates is 13.6 Hz, more than one cycle faster than those considered above.

Block Design. This test correlates with the average frequency of the same order as Similarities, namely 13.5 Hz on the left hemisphere and 13.6 Hz on the right or 13.6 Hz for both hemispheres.

Picture Completion. This is an indisputable test of 'active' intelligence. It correlates with an average frequency of 14.5 Hz on the left, 14.7 Hz on the right and 14.6 Hz for both hemispheres.

Digit Span. This is another indisputable test of 'active' intelligence. It shows lower correlative strength with 8–10 Hz alpha frequency than the first 3 tests of 'passive' intelligence represented by the histograms. It also shows some correlation with 17–19 Hz. The average frequency with which it correlates is 14.0 Hz, 2 Hz higher than for the first 3 tests of 'passive' intelligence.

Arithmetic. This test shows yet another shape of the histogram being definitely favored by frequencies above 12 Hz. It correlates with an average frequency of 14.6 Hz on the left, 14.8 Hz on the right and 14.7 Hz for both hemispheres.

Picture Arrangement. This appears as the most 'active' intelligence exercise. The corresponding histogram shows a 'crescendo' of increasing correlative strength with increasing frequency of the range under consideration. The average frequency with which it correlates is 15.1 Hz, 3 Hz above that correlating with the most typical tests of 'passive' intelligence.

When one scans figure 13/5 one can intuitively confirm the logic of this ascendency, each successive item requiring more 'activation' than the previous one if and when the average correlating frequency increases. This analysis therefore confirms (1) the intrinsic value of the methodology used by *Giannitrapani* and (2) the concept previously advanced for the necessity of 'activation' of certain brain structures in order to be able to carry out certain 'performance' or 'conceptual' aspects of 'active' intelligence. It also implicitly confirms the judicial use by *Wechsler* of different subtests to probe intellectual functions of increasing complexity.

Two other tests of 'active' intelligence, Object Assembly and Coding, have not yet been considered in detail.

Object Assembly. This test showed only 3 significant correlations in the centrotemporal region with 13 Hz, none with 9 or 11 Hz. There was also a significant correlation with 23 Hz beta activity in the left occipital region. There was a great number of borderline negative correlations with theta activity.

Coding. This test shows significant correlations in the occipital regions with theta, 'alpha-plus' and 23-Hz beta activity as well as with 25-Hz beta activity in the central region. There was a negative correlation with slow activity in the centrotemporal regions. This test, as well as Object Assembly, therefore, showed features of both 'active' and 'passive' intelligence.

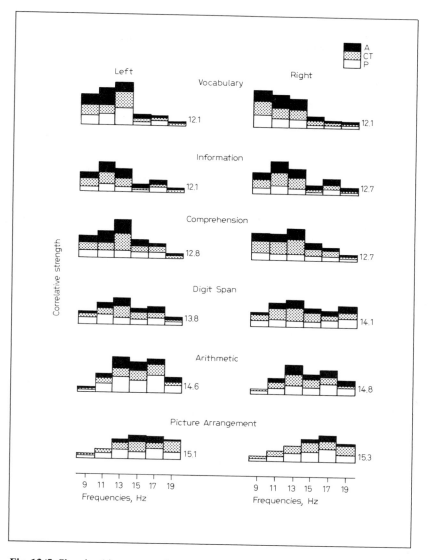

Fig. 13/5. Showing histograms of correlative strength as a function of frequencies for tests of 'passive' (Vocabulary, Information, Comprehension) and 'active' intelligence (Digit Span, Arithmetic, Picture Arrangement) for different regions of the cortex: anterior (A), centrotemporal (CT) and posterior (P = parietal, occipital and posterior temporal). Note that faster frequencies predominate for the last 2 tests of 'active' intelligence. The figures on the graph indicate the average frequency that correlates for either 'passive' or 'active' intelligence subtests.

Regional Differences

It seems to be of prime interest to analyze *Giannitrapani's* data within my frame of reference in terms of regional predominance of the correlative strength of 'alpha-plus' frequencies separately for the anterior, middle and posterior areas of the convexity. For this purpose I introduced the notion of an anterior/posterior ratio. This ratio represents the cumulative correlative strength of these frequencies recorded for the anterior regions divided by the cumulative correlative strength corresponding to these frequencies recorded in the posterior regions. It is considered for each subtest of the WISC (table 13/I). The cumulative correlative strength is obtained by weighing the data in the tables of chapter 9 with the method described at the beginning of the preceding section.

The information represented in this table is remarkable on many accounts. Let me reiterate its direct meaning. If the above ratio is equal to approximately 1 (0.90–1.10) for one particular subtest, this signifies that for the ability of an individual to succeed on this subtest the anterior and posterior regions of the convexity are equally important. If this ratio is significantly above 1.10, it means that the anterior region of the cortex is more important for the achievement on this subtest than the posterior one. If this ratio is significantly below 0.90, it means that the posterior cortex is more important than the anterior for individual achievements on this subtest.

The first impression derived from table 13/I is that the relative importance of the anterior and posterior cortex in the left and right hemispheres are about the same. Both Vocabulary and Information as well as Comprehension scores seem to predominate in the anterior brain, with posterior regions being paramount for successful achievement on the tests involving visual functions, Block Design and Picture Arrangement. Picture Completion for some reason is only marginally favored by the posterior brain just as Arithmetic is. This table therefore underscores the functional importance of the posterior regions for tests involving vision and of the anterior brain for Vocabulary, Information, Comprehension and Similarities. Digit Span relies on both left and right anterior and posterior brains.

Let us now consider the correlative strength of 'alpha-plus' frequencies separately for the entire left and right hemispheres as differentially related to 'passive' and 'active' intelligence (table 13/II). In this table the ratio of total correlative strength of the left over the right hemisphere is considered. The computation is identical to that for table 13/I. When the entire hemispheres are considered, abilities for achievement on Picture Arrangement,

Table 13/I. Ratio of the correlative strength between the anterior and posterior regions of the brain, separately for the 2 hemispheres, for 9 WISC subtests obtained by weighing the dots in tables of chapter 9

	Left	Right		Left	Right
Vocabulary	1.42	1.60	Picture Completion	0.82	0.82
Information	1.70	1.40	Arithmetic	0.85	0.80
Comprehension	1.50	1.40	Block Design	0.68	0.54
Similarities	1.40	1.30	Picture Arrangement	0.28	0.26
Digit Span	1.11	0.91			

Table 13/II. Ratio of the correlative strength between the left and right hemispheres, brain areas and frequencies pooled, for 9 WISC subtests obtained by weighing the dots in tables of chapter 9

Picture Completion	1.80	Vocabulary	1.15	Comprehension	0.98
Similarities	1.46	Block Design	1.15	Information	0.87
Arithmetic	1.25	Picture Arrangement	1.08	Digit Span	0.80

Comprehension and Information depend equally on both hemispheres. For achievement on Picture Completion, Similarities and Arithmetic, the left cortex appears to be paramount. It is important to a lesser degree for Vocabulary and Block Design. For Digit Span, however, the right cortex appears to be more important than the left.

Discussion

The methodology presented by *Giannitrapani*, reconsidered from a different viewpoint in this chapter, sheds new light on the mutual relationship of EEG and intelligence. The notion of 'active' and 'passive' intelligence seems to be useful in considering this relationship in a novel fashion. It appears that the reason we all were stumbling around in the initial search for this relationship was due to the fact that we implicitly considered that theta, alpha, fast, and beta activities were solely characterized by their frequency. Thus, we thought that alpha waves recorded over the occiput were functionally equal to the alpha waves recorded in the central or the frontal regions of the head. Because alpha activity predominates in the occipital regions, we looked for correlations between the occipital alpha rhythm and different aspects of intelligence. With this approach our efforts were doomed to fail, at least partially.

The methodology used by *Giannitrapani,* somewhat modified for this chapter, shows that only certain frequencies of alpha rhythm and only those recorded in certain regions of the brain are correlative with certain subtests of intelligence (mostly 'passive'). No test of 'passive' intelligence correlates with 17-Hz frequency, and no test of 'active' intelligence correlates with 9-Hz rhythm.

The discovery by *Giannitrapani* of the correlative strength of slow activity with intelligence similarly warrants further analysis. Indeed, only subtests of 'passive' intelligence and only slow activity recorded in the posterior half of the head show mutual correlations. Moreover, 'passive' intelligence shows pronounced negative correlations with beta activity. In addition, the present analysis shows that 'active' intelligence correlates mostly with the band of frequencies found between alpha and beta waves, namely 13–23 Hz.

It is important to keep in mind that what is being considered in this chapter is the *ability to succeed* in one or another of the subtests of the WISC, not the *changes actually produced in the EEG during the administration of the test.* Such changes were considered by *Giannitrapani* elsewhere in this book. Thus, the functional significance of these abilities in terms of regional brain wave frequencies emerges. The importance of the frontocentral brain hidden in classical electroencephalography is revealed. The importance of the posterior region for functions involving vision is illustrated. Basic hemispheric differences are disclosed, and EEG significance differentiating between 'active' and 'passive' intelligence is asserted.

Such abilities of the brain are shown to depend on the regional frequency components of the individual electroencephalogram. We do know, however, that an individual may be *trained* to increase his or her achievement in abilities to exercise active intelligence. In other papers we showed that by training one may develop new frequencies in the resting or evoked EEG. We refer the reader to these papers, *Liberson and Ellen* [1960] and *Liberson* [1972].

The results analyzed in this chapter are based on a single experiment carried out on a group of adolescents. Obviously it should be repeated for this and other age groups, including aged individuals with or without mental disease. Then and only then can any conclusions be extended to other populations with any degree of certainty. It is tempting, however, to hypothesize why aged individuals and those with slow EEG abnormalities succeed in tests of 'passive' intelligence and fail in those of 'active' intelligence. Might it be due to the fact that achievement in 'passive' intelligence tests as shown in this chapter depend on slow rhythms and relatively slow alpha activities (in certain regions of the brain) while 'active' intelligence requires the presence of faster rhythms, again in specific regions of the brain? Aged individuals and those with diffuse EEG abnormalities may lack organized fast components of EEG frequencies and thus may not have adequate regional activity required for achievement in 'active' intelligence. They do not lack the slow regional frequencies required to succeed in tests of 'passive' intelligence.

Years ago I formulated the hypothesis that 'active' intelligence depends on structures driven by the subcortex. I still believe in the soundness of this hypothesis. It is obvious, however, that the greater dependence of 'active' intelligence on faster frequency bands (up to 20 Hz) than 'passive' intelligence (correlated with theta and slow alpha activity) demonstrated in this chapter, remains true whether or not the role of the subcortex in this regard is confirmed in the future.

It remains, however, that intuitively the propensity for 'active' intelligence may differ from that of 'passive' intelligence by the intensity of effort that the subject is able or willing to sustain for succeeding in the tests. Indeed, the naive and yet possibly correct notion emerging from examining the requirement for such an effort by different subtests is that they present an increasing intrinsic 'difficulty'. Thus, for example, the Vocabulary subtest requires only the recognition of the meaning of a word without any particular effort. The subject either knows the meaning by previous training or experience or he/she does not. This subtest relates mostly to older learned material. Likewise, Information is either available or not at the time of the testing although it may be related to more recently acquired material. However, success in passing the Digit Span subtest requires an effort of memorizing the presented information then and there. The subject may or may not be willing or able to retain such information. A degree of concentrated attention is required for such a subtest. The same processes of voluntary effort, attention and motivation are required to a graded degree for succeeding in subtests of Arithmetic, Block Design, Picture Completion and Picture Arrangement.

We showed in our studies conducted in the late 1930s that the same subjects who showed a higher achievement in short memory tests did better in tests of prolonged apnea, or duration of a static effort. Later we showed that the propensity for alpha depression under the influence of various types of sensory or intellectual stimulation showed changes with age comparable with those found for 'active' intelligence. One might therefore conceive that a general factor related to motivation, attention and capability for sus-

tained effort is needed for success in subtests of 'active' intelligence, correlated with higher brain wave frequencies in certain regions of the cortex
within the 'alpha-plus' range.

Another factor that may play a latent role in this differentiation is the
time factor. Indeed the tests of 'active' intelligence are generally limited in
time. Without such limitations the subjects might earn higher scores.

Giannitrapani rightly believes that some important information concerning EEG correlations with intelligence may be found not only by
studying the *propensity* of the subject to succeed in one or another test but
also by studying the changes in EEG during the time of the administration
of the test. To our knowledge, *Laugier and Liberson* [1937] were the first to
record EEG during intellectual tasks. We reported at that time that high
theta frequency as well as alpha activity were increasing in the temporofron-
tal regions. *Kennedy* et al. [1949], without citing this initial paper, confirmed our finding and called these waves 'kappa waves'. There was general
uneasiness about the true cerebral origin of kappa waves because of eye
proximity and therefore the possibility of eye-movement artifacts involved
in this activity. *Giannitrapani's* correlative methodology might contribute
to resolving this controversy. Slow activity recorded in the posterior brain is
much less likely to be due to eye movements. It is possible that this activity
reflects the ability of the hippocampus to be 'alerted' during intellectual
effort. We studied analogous phenomena in the past in animals [*Liberson
and Akert,* 1955; *Liberson and Cadilhac,* 1953].

The 'anterior over posterior ratios' computed for this chapter are worth
additional comments. They reveal the predominant importance of the frontal lobes for achievement in some verbal tests such as Vocabulary, Information, Comprehension and Similarities, the latter two being more 'active'
than the first two. However, the exclusive dependence on the frontal lobes
for more typical 'active' intelligence subtests is not revealed by this analysis.
In some subtests such as Block Design and Picture Arrangement the
involvement of the visual function explains the posterior predominance of
correlations. Yet, for Picture Completion, Arithmetic and Digit Span the
anterior and posterior brain regions appear as almost equally important.

Likewise, consideration of the 'left over the right hemispheric ratio'
seems to be revealing. In general, the left hemisphere appears to be more
often indispensable for intellectual effort than the right one. Thus, for
example, for Picture Completion it is almost twice as important as the right
one, and for Similarities and Arithmetic it also appears of predominant
importance. For the rest of the tests, both seem to be equally important

although the right hemisphere claims its ascendance for Digit Span and Symbol Manipulation (see below). This analysis confirms, therefore, the dominance of the left hemisphere for most of the intellectual abilities probed in this experiment.

Since originally I considered as an example of 'active' intelligence the 'conceptual' test of *Shipley* [1940], it was of interest to see how an equivalent test used in the present study would compare with the results of the 'active' subtests of the WISC. The only analogous test to that of *Shipley* that was administered in this study was 'Symbol Manipulation'. Analysis of the data shows that: (1) It correlates mostly negatively with theta activity as some other active WISC intelligence subtests do. (2) It shows a relatively low number of negative correlations (above 0.10) with beta activity (19 Hz). (3) It correlates with relatively high average frequency within the 'alpha-plus' range (14 Hz). (4) It shows a low anterior over posterior ratio (0.64 for the left hemisphere; 0.54 for the right), being comparable to Block Design of the WISC. (5) It shows a very low left over right total hemispheric EEG power ratio (0.71), displaying a greater dependence on the right hemisphere, even more than Digit Span. This indeed is an interesting finding to be investigated further.

All in all, these findings seem to herald an era of new promise and hopefully new achievements in this important area of scientific inquiry.

The Scanning Hypothesis

Finally, a few words concerning chapter 17 of this book. In 1938, almost a half century ago, I formulated a theory that I called the 'law of 3.5' [*Liberson*, 1938]. It stated that all significant frequencies in EEG are multiples of about 3.5 Hz. 'Petit mal discharges' (3.5 Hz); dominant theta activity (6–7 Hz = 2 × 3.5 Hz); alpha rhythm (10.5 Hz = 3 × 3.5 Hz); 'spindles' (14 Hz = 4 × 3.5 Hz) and the peaks of 'beta activity' published then by *Jasper and Andrews* [1937]: 17.5 Hz = 5 × 3.5 Hz; 21 Hz = 6 × 3.5 Hz; 25 Hz = 7 × 3.5 Hz, and 28.5 Hz = 8 × 3.5 Hz.

Since that time additional information has emerged to reinforce my belief in this law [*Liberson*, 1956]. Discovery of the hippocampal theta activity of 6.5- and of positive 6-Hz spikes are 2 of these reinforcing considerations. However, the most revealing contributions have come from the study of EEG power spectral analysis and from the analysis of the mid and long latency components of evoked potentials.

Table 13/III. Relationships between EEG power spectrum frequencies and latencies of somatosensory and auditory evoked potentials

EEG power spectrum rhythms Hz	Reciprocals of freq. ms	Related half-periods ms	After adding 14 ms cond. time to thalamus	6 studies average SS and aud. EPs components ms	Somatosensory potentials component latencies, ms			Auditory evoked potentials component latencies, ms		
					Liberson [1966]	Liberson [1972]	Shagass [1972]	Liberson [1983]	Rapin [1964]	Goff et al. [1977]
29	34	17	31	30	33	30	29.1	–	–	29.0
23	43	21	35	33	–	32	33.4	–	–	32.9
21	48	24	38	39	–	–	–	40	38	40.5
17	59	30	44	49	47	–	47.8	–	49	49.0
13	77	39	53	57	–	–	58.1	–	56	57.0
10	100	50	64	66	62	64	–	–	69	66.0
6.5	142	71	85	80	80	–	73.9	90	80	80.0
5.0	200	100	114	106	115	116	94.1	–	–	106.0
3.4	294	147	161	150	157	132	–	150	151–164	150.0

It is all the more reassuring to find in the data of *Giannitrapani* another confirmation of this law. Indeed, if one considers the 'raw' spectrum and those new components revealed by the analysis of correlations between EEG frequencies and intelligence (tables, chapter 9), one finds the following privileged frequency 'peaks' starting with 10 Hz: 10 Hz (3×3.3 Hz); 13 Hz (4×3.25 Hz); 17 Hz (5×3.4 Hz); 21 Hz, only a 'hillock' (6×3.5 Hz); 23 Hz (7×3.3 Hz) and 29 Hz (9×3.2 Hz). *Giannitrapani's* data deals with frequency bands 2-Hz wide, with a consequent increasing margin of error in the interpretation given above for the higher frequencies. Yet, apparently the 'law of averages' permits one to obtain an impressive concordance of predicted and experimental data. Only 8×3.3 Hz as well as 6.6 Hz (2×3.3 Hz) are missing for inexplicable reasons. On the other hand, an additional peak at 5 Hz emerged. This is the only aberrant number of the series. Yet we believe it to be authentic, representing a subharmonic of a strong 10-Hz frequency (see below).

In order to demonstrate the extension of the 'law' of 3.5 to evoked potentials, table 13/III was formed. In this table the above values were listed in the left column with theta frequency (6.5 Hz) also being listed. The second column transforms these data from a frequency domain to a time domain by taking reciprocals of frequencies. Moreover, because negative and positive peaks are considered for evoked potential latencies, these times are divided by 2, indicating half periods of the corresponding frequencies. If one adds 14 ms, representing the transit time to thalamus to each half period, one obtains values almost equal to the latencies of mid and late components previously published by *Liberson* [1966, 1972, 1983], as well as by *Shagass* [1972], *Rapin* [1964] and *Goff* et al. [1977] for both somatosensory and auditory evoked potential components. The concurrence of values obtained by these two completely independent methodologies is striking [*Liberson and Giannitrapani,* 1984].

Two additional observations must be mentioned: (1) The fact that in both somatosensory and auditory evoked potentials, mid and late components have practically the same latencies. This reinforces the notion that both methodologies reveal the same underlying and often hidden privileged brain wave frequencies, not specifically related to either somatosensory or auditory domains but activated by all the incoming stimuli. (2) The quest for the nature of 3.5-Hz basic frequency must go on. In the past, *Liberson and Cadilhac* [1953] and *Liberson* [1955] mentioned that the time of recovery of excitability following cortical stimulation is of the order of 300–400 ms. *Gastaut* [1952] found a similar time for the recovery curve of the effects of visual stimulation. One may add the intriguing observation that the highest frequency found in our records tends to be 10×3.5 Hz or 35 Hz. 35 Hz happens to be close to the recently mentioned optimal rhythm for auditory stimulation [*Galambos* et al., 1981; *Başar* et al., 1983] as well as to the privileged rhythms mentioned by *Freeman* [1975] for the olfactory system. One must add that it constitutes the highest rhythm of voluntary innervation of muscles when the tetanus is fused.

On the other hand many neurophysiological observations, including those made by *Giannitrapani* in chapter 17 of this book, point to the importance of the 3.5-Hz rhythm. In addition to the examples given there, I may mention that in my old study with *Iavorsky* [*Iavorsky and Liberson*, 1936], we found that this is the frequency of voluntary finger flexion at which the finger movements are no longer perceived as isolated movements but as a global sustained voluntary rhythm.

The scanning hypothesis of *Eccles, McCulloch, Walter* and *Giannitrapani* (see chapter 17) must be considered in relation to these fascinating findings. We are inclined to see in these rhythms an ability of the central nervous system to synchronize incoming information for the different modalities and different brain regions and to act as a filtering resonant system to permit processing of this information, both exogenous and endogenous, at a different rate according to the time requirements of the tasks at hand.

On the conceptual rather than the perceptual level, the basic frequency may be closer to 4 Hz rather than to 3.5 Hz as the studies quoted in chapter 17 suggest. There is therefore an agreement between the approach of *Giannitrapani* and those resulting from my studies. Incidentally, his findings related to the regional activities elicited by mental calculation confirm to an amazing degree the findings of *Laugier and Liberson* [1937] of almost half a century ago. *Giannitrapani's* findings related to the left temporal lobe during listening to a story illustrate the validity of his methodology.

References

Başar, E.; Başar, E.C.; Greitschus, F.; Rosen, B.: 40-Hz component of the auditory evoked potential. Electroenceph. clin. Neurophysiol. *56:* S43 (1983).

Chweitzer, A.; Geblewicz, E.; Liberson, W.T.: Etude de l'électroencéphalogramme humain dans un cas d'intoxication mescalinique. Année Psychol. *27:* 94–119 (1937).

Davis, H.; Davis, P.A.: Action potentials of the brain in normal states of cerebral activity. Archs neurol. Psychiat., Lond. *36:* 1214–1224 (1936).

Freeman, W.Y.: Mass action in the nervous system (Academic Press, New York 1975).

Galambos, R.; Makeig, S.; Talmachoff, P.J.: A 40-Hz auditory potential recorded from the human scalp. Proc. natn. Acad. Sci. USA *78:* 2643–2647 (1981).

Gastaut, H.: Correlations entre le système nerveux végétatif et le système de la vie de relation dans le rhinencéphale. J. Physiol., Paris *44:* 431–470 (1952).

Goff, G.D.; Matsumiya, Y.; Allison, T.; Goff, W.R.: Scalp topography of human somatosensory and auditory evoked potentials. Electroenceph. clin. Neurophysiol. *42:* 57–76 (1977).

Goldstein, L.: Statistical organizational features of the computerized EEG under various behavioral states. Adv. biol. Psychiat., vol. 6, pp. 12–16 (Karger, Basel 1981).

Iavorsky, G.; Liberson, W.T.: Recherches sur le pouvoir de discrimination des mouvements volontaires. Travail Hum. *IV* (1936).

Jasper, H.H.; Andrews, H.L.: Electroencephalography. III. Normal differentiation between occipital and precentral regions in man. Archs Neurol. Psychiat., Lond. *37:* 96–115 (1937).

Kennedy, J.L.; Gottsdanker, R.M.; Armington, J.C.; Gray, F.E.: The kappa rhythm and problem-solving behavior. Electroenceph. clin. Neurophysiol. *1:* 516 (1949).

Laugier, H.; Liberson, W.T.: Contribution à l'étude de l'électroencéphalogramme humain. C.r. Séanc. Soc. Biol. *125:* 13–17 (1937).

Liberson, W.T.: Electroencéphalographie transcranienne chez l'homme. Travail hum. *4:* 303–320 (1936).

Liberson, W.T.: Les données récentes de l'EEG chez l'hommes. Etude différentielle de l'EEG occipital. Biotypologie *6:* 98–134 (1938).

Liberson, W.T.: Recherches biométriques sur les électroencéphalogrammes individuels. Contr. Inst. Biol. Univ. Montréal *9:* 1–19 (1941).

Liberson, W.T.: Ondes électriques du cerveau et intelligence; PhD thesis (mimeographed), Montreal (1950).

Liberson, W.T.: Ondes électriques du cerveau et intelligence chez les malades mentaux. Année psychologique, pp. 677–703 (Presses Universitaires de France, Paris 1951).

Liberson, W.T.: Emotional and psychological factors in epilepsy: physiological background. Am. J. Psychiat. *112:* 91–106 (1955).

Liberson, W.T.: Electroencéphalographie différentielle. Biotypologie *17:* 1–17 (1956).

Liberson, W.T.: Study of evoked potentials in aphasics. Am. J. phys. Med. *45:* 135–142 (1966).

Liberson, W.T.: EEG and intelligence; in Zubin, Jarvik, Psychopathology of mental development, pp. 514–543 (Grune & Stratton, New York 1967).

Liberson, W.T.: Time, space, motivation, memory and decision; in Karczmar, Eccles, Brain and human behavior, pp. 353–376 (Springer, Berlin 1972).

Liberson, W.T.: The law of 3.5 revisited; paper read to EEG Society of French Language, Paris 1983.

Liberson, W.T.; Akert, K.: Hippocampal seizure states in the guinea pig. Electroenceph. clin. Neurophysiol. *7:* 211–222 (1955).

Liberson, W.T.; Cadilhac, J.: Electroshock and rhinencephalic seizure states. Confinia neurol. *13:* 277–286 (1953).

Liberson, W.T.; Ellen, P.: Conditioning of the driven brain wave rhythm in the cortex and the hippocampus of the rat; in Recent advances in biological psychiatry, pp. 158–171 (Grune & Stratton, New York 1960).

Liberson, W.T.; Fried, P.: EEG power spectrum and confusion in the elderly. Electromyogr. clin. Neurophysiol. *21:* 353–367 (1981).

Liberson, W.T.; Giannitrapani, D.: Mid and long frequency components and the law of 3.5. Electromyogr. clin. Neurophysiol. (in press, 1984).

Liberson, W.T.; Liberson, C.W.: EEG records, reaction times, eye movements, respiration and mental content during drowsiness; in Recent advances in biological psychiatry, vol. 8, pp. 295–302 (Plenum Publishing, New York 1966).

Magoun, H.W.: The waking brain; 2nd ed. (Thomas, Springfield 1963).

Rapin, I.: Evoked responses to clicks in a group of children with communication disorders. Ann. N.Y. Acad. Sci. *112:* 182–203 (1964).

Shagass, C.: Evoked brain potentials in psychiatry (Plenum Publishing, New York 1972).

Shipley, W.C.: A self-administering scale for measuring intellectual impairment and deterioration. J. Psychol. *9:* 371–377 (1940).

Strauss, N.; Liberson, W.T.; Meltzer, T.: Electroencephalographic studies: bilateral differences in alpha activity in cases with and without cerebral pathology. J. Mt Sinai Hosp. *9:* 957–962 (1943).

IV Factor Analysis of the EEG

'... If the apparent complexity implied is appalling, what seems to be needed is the courage to face reality. If the next steps do not seem to be clear, then the cure is more knowledge – knowledge concerning the whole list of intellectual factors, their relations to complex mental functioning, and their relations to everyday behavior.'
J.P. Guilford

14 History of EEG Factor Analysis Studies

'Let us press on with the serious, persistent, and if necessary daring, exploration of the thought processes, by all available means.'
D.O. Hebb

The EEG technique was born from a pragmatic basis and developed through pragmatic correlations between visually detectable electrophysiological parameters and behavior or pathology. For further development, the field needed an understanding of the mechanisms governing these correlations. A necessary foundation for the understanding of these mechanisms was an understanding of the nature of the EEG.

Progress in EEG development has been hampered by current electrophysiological knowledge which is basically unequipped to handle the complexity of a signal which, given its voltage, it is safe to assume is the resultant of the activity of millions of cells. This lack of understanding of the mechanism underlying the EEG phenomenon has kept many scientists from entering the field and has kept others from asking complex questions such as whether these impulses reflected in some way higher cortical functions.

There have been some efforts, however, to improve upon the current understanding of EEG parameters from the original eyeballing method [*Walter*, 1963; *Walter and Adey*, 1966; *Dumermuth* et al., 1971; *Hjorth*, 1970; *Oldenbürger and Becker*, 1975; *Burger*, 1980].

In a few cases the factor analysis methodology was employed. These studies can be subdivided into 4 groups depending upon the purpose for which the factor analysis technique was utilized.

One group of studies was purely theoretical-methodological [*Joseph and Remond*, 1971; *Walter*, 1973; *Oldenbürger* et al., 1975; *Holoubková* et al., 1978]. Their purpose was to stimulate thinking and the possibility of improving the set of data available in order to draw better conclusions from the available parameters.

A second group of studies, motivated by the obvious redundancy of the eyeballing method, factor analyzed broad frequency bands which reproduced traditional EEG broad band categories and attempted to answer questions addressed by either the clinical or the experimental electroencephalographer. Among these studies, the EEG changes due to different behavioral states were addressed by *Walter* et al. [1967]; ontogenetic changes in EEG by *Chavance* et al. [1975], *Chavance and Samson-Dolfuss* [1978], *Pratusevich* et al. [1981], *Gasser* et al. [1983a, b]. The cerebral organic pathology question was addressed by *Faber* et al. [1975], *Zhirmunskaya* et al. [1979]; changes due to psychotropic drug effects by *Faber* et al. [1974], *Etevenon* [1975], *Burger and Lairy* [1978]; changes due to toxic inhalation as well as to psychotropic drug effects by *Dvořák* et al. [1981]; changes due to hemodialysis by *Spehr* et al. [1977]; the EEG in juvenile delinquents by *Ishihara and Yoshii* [1972]; characteristics of sleep EEG in children by *Burger and Catani* [1981]; mental retardation by *Gasser* et al. [1983a, b]; and intelligence by *Gasser* et al. [1983c].

A third group of studies was stimulated by the clinicians' need for a better clinical tool and attempted to verify through factor analysis the existing eyeball-defined frequency bands (e.g. alpha, beta, delta, theta). Among these were *Defayolle and Dinand* [1974]; *Dymond* et al. [1978]; *Hermann* et al. [1978a, b].

All of these investigators performed factor analysis of either one or 2 EEG derivations, using from 1 to 4 conditions. Their attempts to verify the traditional clinical EEG frequency bands met with mixed success. While the findings seem to support, in general, the traditional EEG frequency bands, there were several points of variance, partly due to different populations, different conditions and different EEG derivations. *Oldenbürger and Becker* [1975] cautioned against using classical frequency bands which were based upon unproven assumptions. They argued from their limited vantage point, i.e. a study based on the analysis of one derivation, against the dangers of hypothesizing clusters from factor analyses.

A fourth group of studies did not start with an a priori conviction of the validity of the eyeball-determined frequency bands and preferred to explore the spectrum of frequencies unfettered by preconceptions. These studies used narrow band frequency analysis and factor analysis to their full potential, namely to investigate what relationship existed between the full spectrum of EEG frequencies, what degree of independence existed between individual frequencies and under what behavioral states these relationships changed.

Among these studies, *Larsen* [1969] explored the physiological sources of covariation and their changes under different conditions. Again only 1 derivation (C_z-O_1) was used. *Nebylitsin and Aleksandrova* [1971] investigated dispersion parameters of frontal and occipital EEG in one condition and found that the stability and periodicity of the EEG separated into 2 factors, each representing the 2 derivations studied. *Löwenhard* [1973], using a repetitive measure design from one bipolar derivation (C_4-O_2), observed a factor structure having a greater degree of complexity than the traditional broad EEG frequency band, and *Elmgren and Löwenhard* [1973], using 2 bipolar derivations (C_4-O_2 and C_3-O_1), had similar results. *Wilhelm and Becker* [1975], from a temporal-occipital derivation, studied emotional states with this technique; *Rösler* [1975], with a left occipital derivation and 6 stimulus situations, studied personality variables; and *Bente* [1979], again from one derivation (bioccipital), studied changes in psychotropic medication.

Among all of these studies, those investigators who attempted to verify traditional broad band EEG frequencies were frustrated by not being able to fully verify the traditional frequency bands which by common custom were regarded not as theoretical constructs but as facts. Those who did not make these assumptions about the reality of these bands found themselves restricted to merely describing their findings.

One additional difficulty that these investigators encountered was the abstruse nature of the factor analysis technique, not readily translatable into a construct having physiological meaning, so that many of these investigators found themselves charting hyperspace, eigen values and other sophisticated parameters not yet being a part of a body of knowledge to which the neurophysiologists or clinicians were accustomed. Since the studies were limited to 1 or 2 derivations, for the most part involving occipital areas, and since these were pioneering studies, there was a tendency to overgeneralize the findings by implying the representativeness of the factor structures.

Consider the fact that these were attempts at data reduction, and in many ways these investigators had succeeded in reducing on a mathematical basis the number of descriptors necessary for describing a function, but the resultant description had the potential of being more accurate and of describing parameters heretofore left undescribed as they were unavailable with the visual inspection of the EEG. The resultant then was data proliferation rather than data reduction, and these problems were present even while relegating the analysis to 1 or 2 scalp areas. The topographic problems of multiple channel representation of these factors were yet to be solved.

Dolce and Decker [1975] performed a full narrow band spectral analysis of the EEG from 0 to 30 Hz in 8 derivations under different conditions of stimulation. They came closest to utilizing the full potential of factor analysis, performing a study in which the interplay of different brain areas was studied.

Finally, *Giannitrapani* [1980, 1982], due to the availability of methods for handling multiple EEG channels concomitantly, studied 16 derivations during 8 different conditions in 16 frequency bands and attempted to solve the staggering problem of displaying such a vast number of data points in a manner comprehensible to the brain investigator, as will be seen in the following chapters.

References

Bente, D.: Die faktorenanalytische Verarbeitung spektraler EEG-Daten: Auswertungsstrategien und pharmakoelektroenzephalographische Anwendungsbeispiele. Z. EEG-EMG *10:* 207–213 (1979).

Burger, D.: Analysis of electrophysiological signals: a comparative study of two algorithms. Comput. Biomed. Res. *13:* 73–86 (1980).

Burger, D.; Catani, P.: Analyse multifactorielle des variables EEG et polygraphiques lors de l'endormissement chez l'enfant. Revue EEG Neurophysiol. *11:* 59–67 (1981).

Burger, D.; Lairy, G.C.: Multivariate analysis of drug-effects on electrophysiological signals in man. Neuropharmacology *17:* 891–904 (1978).

Chavance, M.; Samson-Dollfus, D.: Analyse spectrale de l'EEG de l'enfant normal entre 6 et 16 ans: choix et validation des paramètres les plus informationnels. Electroenceph. clin. Neurophysiol. *45:* 767–776 (1978).

Chavance, M.; Samson-Dollfus, D.; Goldberg, P.: Spectral analysis and statistical description of EEG of normal children from 10 to 12 years old; in Matejcek, Schenk, Quantitative analysis of the EEG. Proc. Study Group for EEG-Methodology, Jongny-sur-Vevey 1975, pp. 589–599.

Defayolle, M.; Dinand, J.P.: Application de l'analyse factorielle à l'étude de la structure de l'EEG. Electroenceph. clin. Neurophysiol. *36:* 319–322 (1974).

Dolce, G.; Decker, H.: Application of multivariate statistical methods in analysis of spectral values of the EEG. CEAN, computerized EEG analysis, pp. 157–171 (Fischer, Stuttgart 1975).

Dumermuth, G.; Huber, P.J.; Kleiner, B.; Gasser, T.: Analysis of the interrrelations between frequency bands of the EEG by means of the bispectrum. A preliminary study. Electroenceph. clin. Neurophysiol. *31:* 137–148 (1971).

Dvořák, J.; Formánek, J.; Kubát, J.; Plevová, J.; Vaničková, M.; Fireš, M.; Anděl, J.; Cipra, T.; Tomášek, L.; Prášková, Z.; Holoubková, E.; Fabián, Z.: Analysis of the time series of the EEG frequency spectra and of EEG spectral power densities. Activitas nerv. sup. *23:* 157–168 (1981).

Dymond, A.M.; Coger, R.W.; Serafetinides, E.A.: Prepocessing by factor analysis of centro-occipital EEG power and asymmetry from three subject groups. Ann. Biomed. Eng. 6: 108–116 (1978).

Elmgren, J.; Löwenhard, P.: Un analisis factorial del EEG humano. Revta Psicol. gen. aplic. 28: 255–271 (1973).

Etevenon, P.: CEAN parameters in neuropsychopharmacology. CEAN, computerized EEG analysis, pp. 236–250 (Fischer, Stuttgart 1975).

Faber, J.; Tošovský, J.; Hynek, K.: Factor analysis of EEG of healthy subjects given no drugs and a combination of diazepam and methylphenidate. Activitas nerv. sup. 16: 258–259 (1974).

Faber, J.; Tošovský, J.; Hynek, K.; Dušek, J.: Factor analysis of EEG in healthy and diseased subjects. Activitas nerv. sup. 17: 139–143 (1975).

Gasser, T.; Möcks, J.; Bächer, P.: Topographic factor analysis of the EEG with applications to development and to mental retardation. Electroenceph. clin. Neurophysiol. 55: 445–463 (1983a).

Gasser, T.; Möcks, J.; Lenard, H.G.; Bächer, P.; Verleger, R.: The EEG of mildly retarded children: developmental, classificatory, and topographic aspects. Electroenceph. clin. Neurophysiol. 55: 131–144 (1983b).

Gasser, T.; Lucadou-Müller, I. von; Verleger, R.; Bächer, P.: Correlating EEG and IQ: a new look at an old problem using computerized EEG parameters. Electroenceph. clin. Neurophysiol. 55: 493–504 (1983c).

Giannitrapani, D.: EEG factors derived through spectral analysis. Soc. Neurosci., Abstracts, 1980, p. 566.

Giannitrapani, D.: Localization of language and arithmetic functions via EEG factor analysis. Res. Commun. psychol. psychiat. Behav. 7: 39–55 (1982).

Herrmann, W.M.; Fichte, K.; Kubicki, S.: Mathematische Rationale für die klinischen EEG-Frequenzbänder. 1. Faktorenanalyse mit EEG-Powerspektralschätzungen zur Definition von Frequenzbändern. Z. EEG-EMG 9: 146–154 (1978a).

Herrmann, W.M.; Fichte, K.; Kubicki, S.: Mathematische Rationale für die klinischen EEG-Frequenzbänder. 2. Stabilität der Faktorenstruktur bei zwei Länderstichproben und Messwiederholungen unter Plazebo. Z. EEG-EMG 9: 200–205 (1978b).

Hjorth, B.: EEG analysis based on time domain properties. EEG clin. Neurophysiol. 29: 306–310 (1970).

Holoubková, E.; Roth, Z.; Formánek, J.: Extension of a computer program for factor analysis of the time series of EEG frequency spectra. Activitas nerv. sup. 20: 28–30 (1978).

Ishihara, T.; Yoshii, N.: Multivariate analytic study of EEG and mental activity in juvenile delinquents. Electroenceph. clin. Neurophysiol. 33: 71–80 (1972).

Joseph, J.P.; Remond, A.: Factorial analysis of EEG rhythms. Electroenceph. clin. Neurophysiol. 30: 369–370 (1971).

Larsen, L.E.: An analysis of the intercorrelations among spectral amplitudes in the EEG: a generator study. IEEE Trans. biomed. Engng BME 16: 23–26 (1969).

Löwenhard, P.: P factor analysis of single EEG recordings. Göteborg Psychol. Rep. 3: 1–14 (1973).

Nebylitsin, V.D.; Aleksandrova, N.J.: Factor analysis of relationship between the EEG quantitative parameters in the frontal and occipital lobes as related to the problem of general properties of the nervous system. Fiziol. Zh. SSSR 57: 1577–1586 (1971).

Oldenbürger, H.-A.; Becker, D.: Are there clusters of frequencies in power spectra of EEG? How to find and prove them statistically; in Matejcek, Schenk, Quantitative analysis of the EEG. Proc. Study Group for EEG Methodology, Jongny-sur-Vevey 1975, pp. 601–611.

Oldenbürger, H.-A.; Becker, D.; Steyer, R.: On the methodology of the comparison of data reduction methods in EEG: a programmatic outline; in Matejcek, Schenk, Quantitative analysis of the EEG. Proc. Study Group for EEG Methodology, Jongny-sur-Vevey 1975, pp. 613–622.

Pratusevich, Y.M.; Solov'ev, A.V.; Kvasov, G.I.: Utilization of factor analysis for the evaluation of ontogenetic and functional changes in the electrical activity of the brain. J. Hyg. Epid. Microbiol. Immunol. *25:* 259–269 (1981).

Rösler, F.: Die Abhängigkeit des Elektroenzephalogramms von den Persönlichkeitsdimensionen E und N sensu Eysenck und unterschiedlich aktivierenden Situationen. Z. exp. angew. Psychol. *XXII:* 630–667 (1975).

Spehr, W.; Sartorious, H.; Berglund, K.; Hjorth, B.; Kablitz, C.; Plog, U.; Wiedemann, P.H.; Zapp, K.: EEG and haemodialysis, a structural survey of EEG spectral analysis, Hjorth's EEG descriptors, blood variables and psychological data. Electroenceph. clin. Neurophysiol. *43:* 787–797 (1977).

Walter, D.O.: Spectral analysis for electroencephalograms: mathematical determination of neurophysiological relationships from records of limited duration. Expl Neurol. *8:* 155–181 (1963).

Walter, D.O.: Two classes of feature-extracting processes; in Kellaway, Petersén, Automation of clinical electroencephalography, pp. 295–299 (Raven Press, New York 1973).

Walter, D.O.; Adey, W.R.: Linear and nonlinear mechanisms of brainwave generation. Ann. N.Y. Acad. Sci. *128:* 772–780 (1966).

Walter, D.O.; Rhodes, J.M.; Adey, W.R.: Discriminating among states of consciousness by EEG measurements. A study of four subjects. Electroenceph. clin. Neurophysiol. *22:* 22–29 (1967).

Wilhelm, H.; Becker, D.: EEG-Veränderungen bei subliminaler Darbietung emotionell unterschiedlich wirksamer Wörter; in Tack, Bericht über den 29. Kongr. der Deutschen Ges. f. Psychologie, Salzburg 1974, vol. 1, pp. 126–127 (Verlag für Psychologie, Göttingen 1975).

Zhirmunskaya, E.A.; Fomicheva, G.P.; Bukhshtaber, V.M.; Maslov, V.K.; Veksler, A.S.; Zelen'yuk, E.A.: Use of method of multidimensional statistical analysis of the EEG to assess the state of cerebral neurodynamics. Hum. Physiol. *5:* 447–455 (1979).

15 Functional Role of EEG Frequencies

'... an enchanted loom where millions of flashing shuttles
weave a dissolving pattern, always a meaningful pattern
though never an abiding one; ...'
Sir *Charles Sherrington,* on the brain

The following factor analyses were undertaken to determine the factor structure of steady-state EEG under specific conditions of stimulation and to compare the frequency components characteristic of each condition with those inferred as having a role in specific intellectual functions as discussed in the preceding chapters. The 8 conditions described in the method chapter (chapter 3) were used. They consisted of 2 resting conditions, Resting I at the beginning and Resting II at the end of the experiment; 3 auditory conditions, Noise (white noise), Music and Voice; 1 mental arithmetic condition, Arithmetic, and 2 open-eyes conditions, Vision (patterned vision) and Diffuse (diffuse vision).

The subject sample, identical to that in chapters 5 and 7–13 consisted of 56 right-preferent subjects. The EEG samples were also those used in those analyses except that in addition the 33-Hz band was also studied. To recapitulate, for each condition Fast Fourier analysis was performed on 8 s of EEG to obtain power density estimates for each of 17 bands from 0 to 34 Hz, each 2-Hz wide. A total of 272 variables was thus obtained and used in the factor analyses.

A principal component analysis with Varimax rotation was performed for each of the 8 conditions via BMD program P4M [*Frane and Jennrich,* 1979]. Initially about 30 factors were obtained, but subsequently the analyses were restricted to 10 factors which seemed to delineate the main frequency groups. Principal component analyses [cf. *Harman,* 1967] and direct quartimin oblique analyses [*Jennrich and Sampson,* 1966] were also performed, but of the 3, Varimax rotation seemed to yield the more meaningful results. Since oblique analysis was almost identical to the Varimax rotation as already observed by *Löwenhard* [1973] and did not furnish additional information, the discussion is restricted to the Varimax rotation factors which are orthogonal, i.e. completely independent from each other.

Table 15/I summarizes the distribution of the factors in relation to traditional EEG categories. At first, headings of the EEG frequencies are listed in order of increasing frequency. The following headings are those of homologously symmetrical EEG activity in specific brain areas after which are listed the headings of EEG activity which are homologously asymmetrical. The table shows for the different conditions a certain degree of similarity and a certain degree of independence which will be discussed here.

Figures 15/1–15/8 show in a schematic form the distribution of factor loadings of the first 9 factors for each of the 8 conditions. The tenth factor is not shown in these figures for ease of display but will be discussed whenever relevant.

Table 15/I. Summary of the factors obtained for each of the 8 conditions. Each column contains the 10 factors for each analysis. Each row contains the factors that can be grouped under the given EEG category

	Resting I	Noise	Music	Voice	Arith-metic	Vision	Diffuse	Resting II
1–3 Hz			1			10	7	9
5–9 Hz	3	4	6, 8	3	3	2	3	2
11 Hz	6	6	5	6			5	4
11, 13 Hz						5		
13–15 Hz	5	9			7, 8	9		7
13, 23 Hz			4	4			6	
9, 15, 17 Hz						4		
15–17 Hz	8			5				
19–33 Hz						1		
27 Hz central					6			
29 Hz	2	3	2	1	2	3	2	1
Anterior slow	9	8	10	7	9, 10	6	4	5
Posterior slow		2			5			
Prefrontal fast	7	5	7	8	4			6
Anterior fast			3					
Post-temporal fast								3
Occipital fast	4	7					8	
Right anterior				9				8
Right temporal and lateral frontal		1			1		1	
Left temporal fast	1		9	2				10
Miscellaneous	10	10		10		7, 8	9, 10	

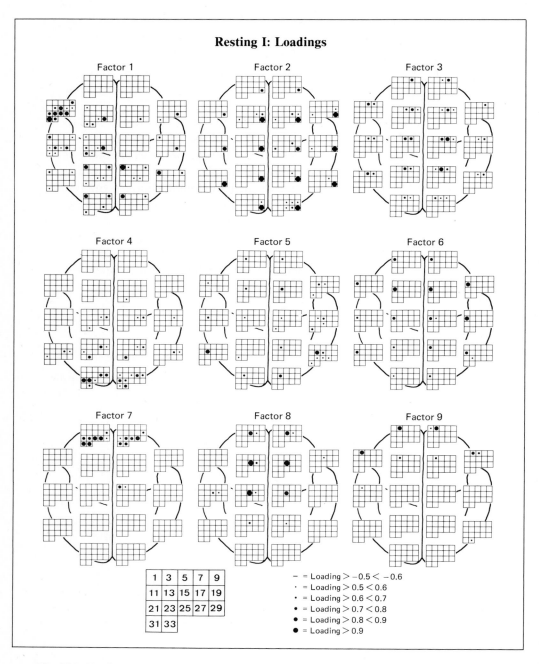

Fig. 15/1. Resting I: topographic representation of the distribution and magnitude of loadings for the first 9 factors. Insert identifies the frequency bands to which the loadings in the figure refer.

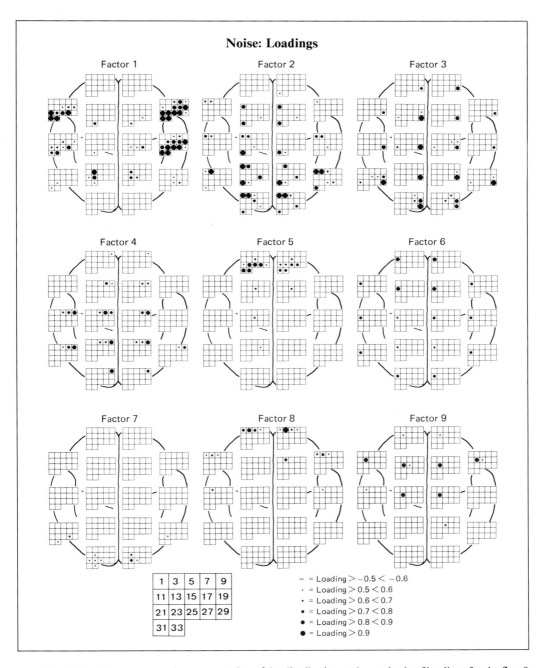

Fig. 15/2. Noise: topographic representation of the distribution and magnitude of loadings for the first 9 factors. Insert identifies the frequency bands to which the loadings in the figure refer.

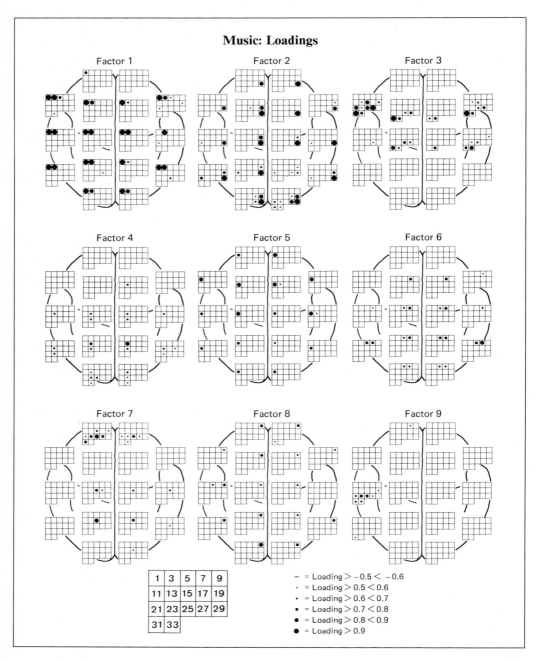

Fig. 15/3. Music: topographic representation of the distribution and magnitude of loadings for the first 9 factors. Insert identifies the frequency bands to which the loadings in the figure refer.

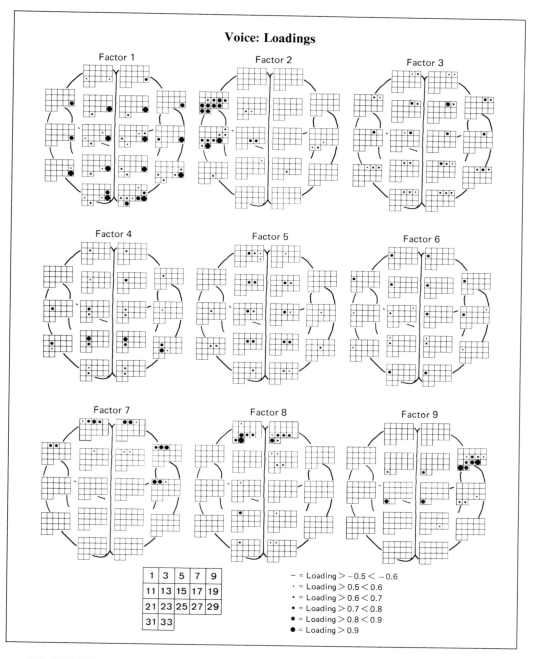

Fig. 15/4. Voice: topographic representation of the distribution and magnitude of loadings for the first 9 factors. Insert identifies the frequency bands to which the loadings in the figure refer.

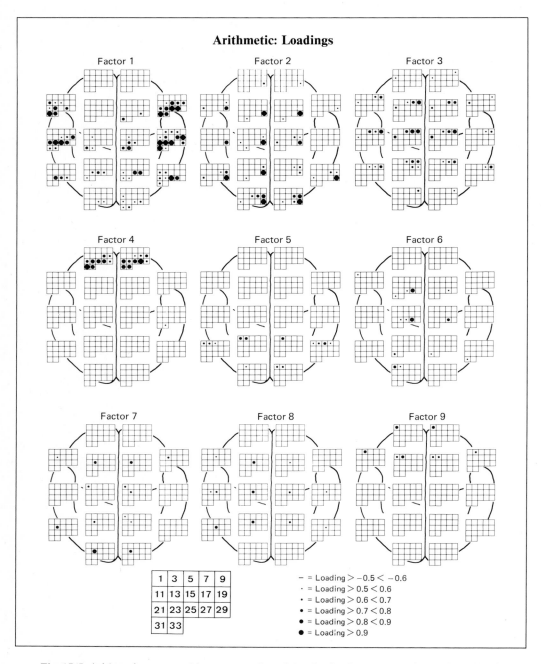

Fig. 15/5. Arithmetic: topographic representation of the distribution and magnitude of loadings for the first 9 factors. Insert identifies the frequency bands to which the loadings in the figure refer.

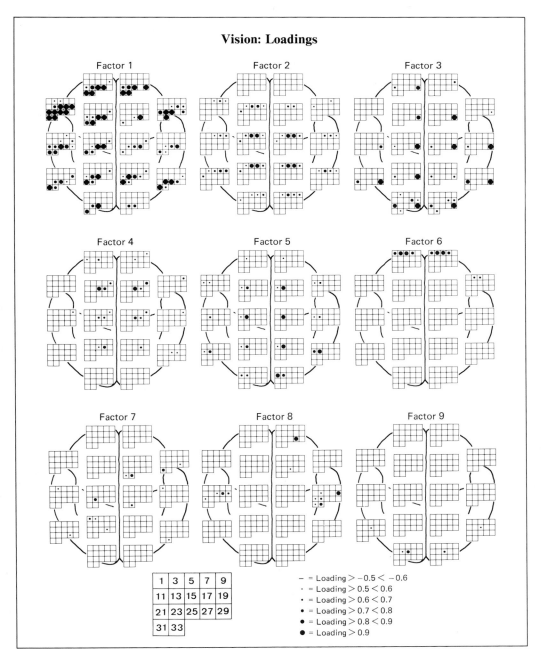

Fig. 15/6. Vision: topographic representation of the distribution and magnitude of loadings for the first 9 factors. Insert identifies the frequency bands to which the loadings in the figure refer.

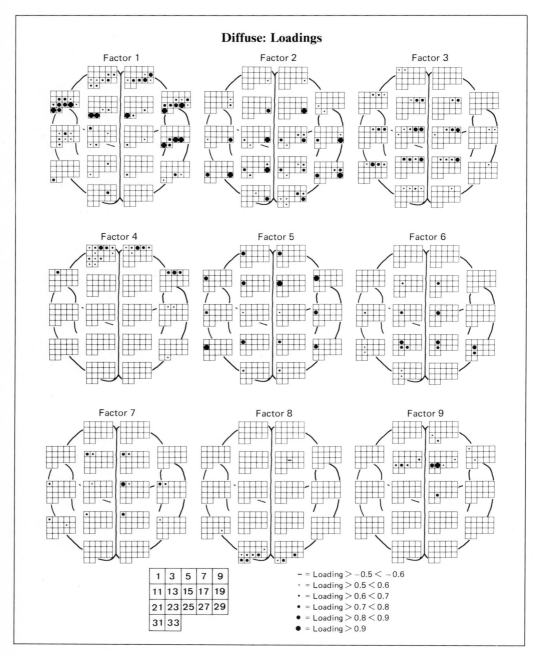

Fig. 15/7. Diffuse: topographic representation of the distribution and magnitude of loadings for the first 9 factors. Insert identifies the frequency bands to which the loadings in the figure refer.

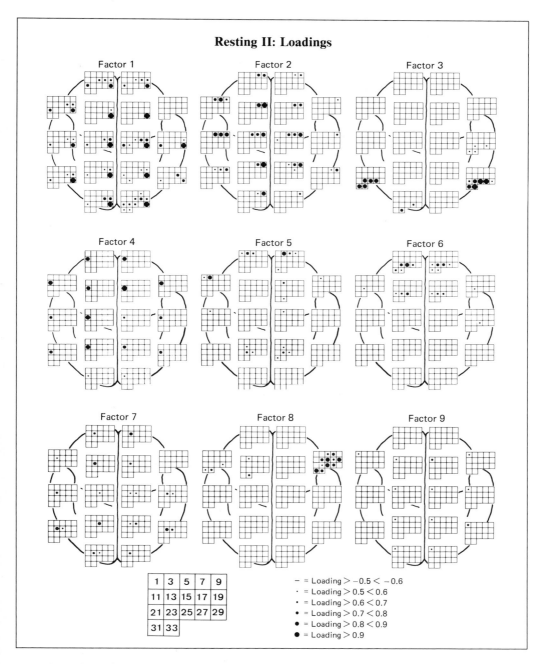

Fig. 15/8. Resting II: topographic representation of the distribution and magnitude of loadings for the first 9 factors. Insert identifies the frequency bands to which the loadings in the figure refer.

Table 15/II. Proportion of the total variance accounted for by each of the 10 factors for each of the analyses performed for the 8 conditions

Factor	Resting I	Noise	Music	Voice	Arith-metic	Vision	Diffuse	Resting II
1	0.138	0.164	0.126	0.125	0.184	0.266	0.154	0.148
2	0.098	0.142	0.120	0.094	0.110	0.110	0.114	0.096
3	0.087	0.105	0.093	0.078	0.099	0.097	0.092	0.065
4	0.083	0.068	0.067	0.067	0.061	0.063	0.063	0.060
5	0.072	0.056	0.061	0.066	0.051	0.059	0.057	0.055
6	0.058	0.051	0.057	0.065	0.049	0.043	0.052	0.053
7	0.055	0.044	0.056	0.057	0.046	0.038	0.048	0.052
8	0.047	0.043	0.054	0.054	0.040	0.035	0.040	0.049
9	0.041	0.041	0.034	0.053	0.037	0.029	0.040	0.038
10	0.035	0.033	0.033	0.034	0.035	0.028	0.032	0.036
Cumulative proportion of variance	0.714	0.747	0.701	0.693	0.712	0.768	0.692	0.652

Table 15/II shows the variance accounted for by each factor for each of the 8 conditions as well as the cumulative proportion of variance accounted for by the 10 factors, separately for each condition.

Factors Organized around EEG Frequencies

1–3 Hz. In this frequency range 4 factors appear. While the factor for Music is the first factor (which in this analysis accounts for 13% of the variance), the other 3 factors are of much less importance and account for a much more limited portion of the variance. Vision factor 10 (not shown) accounts for only 3% of the variance (table 15/II); Diffuse vision factor 7 (fig. 15/7) accounts for 5% of the variance; and Resting II factor 9 (fig. 15/8) accounts for 4% of the variance in their respective analyses. Music factor 1 (fig. 15/3), therefore, stands alone and will be interpreted here as representing a function unrelated to the function represented by the other 3 factors.

In the Music condition the stimulus was Tschaikovsky's *Marche Miniature* with a rhythm of 2/s which could have produced a corresponding brain activity which would have loaded the 2 adjacent frequency bands of 0–2 and 2–4 Hz. This hypothesis was tested by producing, with a synthesizer, rhythms of different frequencies. Spectral peaks in the corresponding frequencies were found in the EEG. It was concluded that this was a specific case of what was heretofore known as EEG driving. If these 2 sets of events belong to the same family of phenomena, the possibility arises that for a stimulus to enter the brain for processing and eventually acquiring meaning, it needs to first be duplicated in its frequency components. Since in the case of the march the rhythm is repetitive, the frequency becomes of such strength that it is easily identifiable as a factor. With nonrepetitive stimuli it is more difficult to demonstrate the mimicking hypothesis because of the signal being buried in the EEG noise. Studies are in progress to verify this hypothesis, especially in the speech frequency range which so far has been regarded as being outside the EEG frequency range.

5–9 Hz. In this frequency range each condition contributed at least one factor. The ubiquitousness of this frequency range and the relatively small range in the percentage of variance accounted for make it difficult to relate this factor to any specific condition except perhaps the Music condition in which this frequency range is divided into 2 factors (fig. 15/3), factor 6 comprising the 5- and 7-Hz frequency and factor 8 comprising the 9-Hz frequency. The relevance of the separation of this frequency range in the Music condition cannot be interpreted at this time.

11 and 11–13 Hz. The 11-Hz activity which included the dominant alpha band for this group of subjects also shows a ubiquitous presence except for Arithmetic and the patterned Vision conditions. Whenever present, this frequency, even though including dominant alpha, surprisingly accounts for less variance than the 5- to 9-Hz frequency band. Previous evidence indicated that alpha *desynchronized* under a varied array of conditions, and the qualitative difference of this desynchronization was difficult to ascertain.

By factoring out the different frequency components in the present analysis of the data, it can be observed that in the Arithmetic condition the distribution of dominant alpha completely disappears. In the patterned Vision condition it is minimized but appears as a component of the 13-Hz activity (factor 5, fig. 15/6), while in the Diffuse vision condition the alpha activity is basically unaffected.

From this observation it can be concluded that the Arithmetic condition, among the range of conditions studied, is unique in its affecting dominant alpha activity. The Arithmetic condition is the only condition of this group in which the subject is required to actively perform a task. Since there are other differences between the Arithmetic condition and the other conditions, isolation of the function responsible for this alpha desynchronization remains to be studied.

13–15 Hz. A factor representing this frequency range is present in the Resting I and II conditions (fig. 15/1, 15/8) in practically identical form. It is also present in the Noise condition (fig. 15/2) with an anterior distribution and in the patterned Vision condition (fig. 15/6) with a post-temporal-occipital distribution. The most interesting feature here is the separation of this range in the mental Arithmetic condition into 2 factors (fig. 15/5), factors 7 and 8. Factor 7 is loaded basically on the 13-Hz band while factor 8 is loaded on the 15-Hz band.

As demonstrated in chapter 9, the 13- and 15-Hz activities were shown to be related to mental Arithmetic, and it is of interest here to show that during the performance of mental Arithmetic, this frequency range separates into 2 individual factors, possibly presiding over the performance of separate functions of this task.

13, 23 Hz. These 2 frequencies are organized in a specific factor under the Music, Voice and Diffuse vision conditions. In chapters 9 and 12 it was shown that the presence of 13-Hz activity and to a lesser extent 23-Hz activity were related to verbal intelligence. The fact that similar factors with somewhat equal loading occur not only for Voice (fig. 15/4) but also for Music (fig. 15/3) and Diffuse vision (fig. 15/7) is not quite understood.

9, 15, 17 Hz. This particular frequency grouping with a frontal distribution is not interpreted at this time. It should be noted, however, that patterned Vision is the only condition in which 9-Hz activity is divided between 2 factors (fig. 15/6). Factor 2 includes 9-Hz activity for a broad spectrum of areas except the prefrontal and especially in the parietal and post-temporal derivations, while factor 4, also having broad distribution, is loaded specifically in the right frontal and right lateral frontal areas, areas which were absent in the loadings of factor 2. It will be interesting to determine the functional significance of this separation and whether this type of analysis of frequency distribution throughout brain areas can be used to infer the presence of generators or the changes in patterns of generation under different functional states.

15–17 Hz. The presence of these fast frequencies in the Resting I condition (fig. 15/1) is being interpreted as evidence that in this condition the subject is not really at rest but is quite tense, maybe apprehensive about what is expected of him. Other factors will corroborate this interpretation. The presence of this factor in the Voice condition factor 5 (fig. 15/4) is in concordance with some of the evidence in chapter 12 relating to the presence of these faster frequencies in some of the verbal subtests of the Wechsler Intelligence Scale for Children (WISC).

19–33 Hz. Factor 1 of the patterned Vision condition (fig. 15/6) shows a unique distribution of activity found only in this condition. The frequencies are strong in all brain areas with perhaps an homologous asymmetry with greater loading in the left lateral frontal area. The frequency range is quite broad and can be compared with factor 1 of the Diffuse vision condition (fig. 15/7) which will be discussed later because of its primarily right-sided distribution.

The opposite asymmetry in these 2 conditions can be discussed in the context of the Voice condition with its asymmetry favoring the left side in the lateral frontal and temporal areas in these frequencies (Voice factor 2, fig. 15/4), pointing to a differential role of the left and right temporal and lateral frontal areas. It could be concluded that the left temporal and lateral frontal areas preside over the processing of stimuli that are meaningful while the right side plays a stronger role when the stimuli do not have meaning or figure. This subject will be discussed in greater detail in chapter 16.

27-Hz Central. A factor loaded primarily on 27 Hz is only present in Arithmetic factor 6 (fig. 15/5). The distribution is primarily frontal and central, and the functional significance of this factor is not interpretable at this time except for its relation to the processing of numerical information.

29 Hz. This ubiquitous frequency band is one of the strongest factors among all of the conditions studied. In previous research [*Giannitrapani and Kayton,* 1974] this frequency was shown to be stronger in schizophrenics as compared to normals, but it was also shown to be stronger in the left-handed group as compared with the right-handed [*Giannitrapani,* 1979a] and also in girls as compared with boys [*Giannitrapani,* 1974, 1979b, 1981, 1982]. It is difficult to interpret at this time the particular role the 29-Hz activity has, but it is relevant to note that it is a relatively unknown frequency that has not been studied primarily because of its low amplitude among the fast frequencies and is therefore undetectable in the visual inspection of the EEG.

Factors Organized around Brain Regions

Anterior Slow. The group of factors subsumed under this category shows at least one representative in each of the conditions tested, but they may not represent a unitary function. The factors containing loadings in the

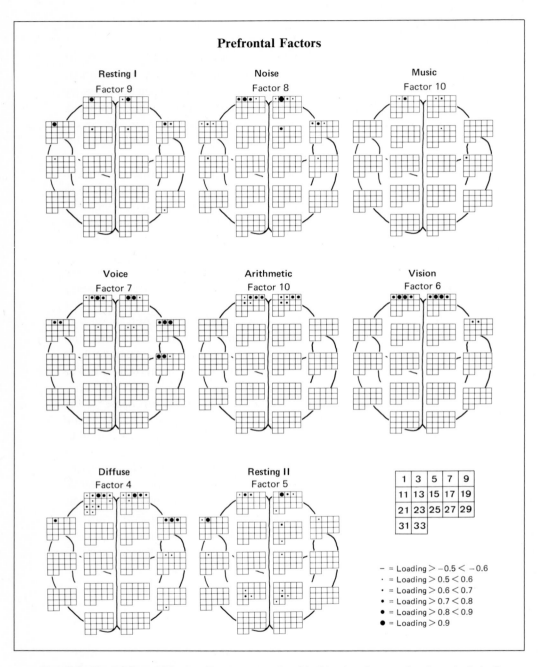

Fig. 15/9. The Prefrontal Factors, shown separately with the other factors of each analysis in figures 15/1–15/8, are regrouped to facilitate comparison.

prefrontal areas in the slow frequency range are regrouped for clarity in figure 15/9. There is a great range of distributions, both in the derivations affected and in frequencies. For instance, in Music factor 10 the distribution is prefrontal in the 3- to 5-Hz band. In Resting I factor 9 the distribution is prefrontal, frontal and lateral frontal in frequencies 1 and 3. The same pattern is shown in Arithmetic factor 9 (fig. 15/5), but Arithmetic factor 10 (fig. 15/9) shows distribution from 3 to 15 Hz in the prefrontal derivations alone.

Three possible hypotheses are being formulated for the existence of prefrontal slow activity. The first is that a portion of these factors may be attributable to eye-movement artifacts which are known to appear in the slow frequency bands and, in support of this hypothesis, factor 4 of the Diffuse vision condition is the factor having the highest rank among all factors in this category. It is known that random eye movements generally increase in the Diffuse vision condition.

The second hypothesis deals with the possibility that prefrontal slow activity occurs during momentary pauses while engaging in mental activity. As described in the method section, the Arithmetic condition consisted of sequential subtractions, namely subtracting 7 from 100, the serial subtractions being performed silently. In the raw record for some subjects, it was noted that there was a periodic volley of slow activity which would occur during the performance of this task, and these volleys could be hypothesized to be related to the achievement of interim solutions, i.e. performing one subtraction and arriving at a result, pausing momentarily to fix on that result and then engaging in the following subtraction. Arithmetic factor 10 shows a unique distribution of frequencies (the only factor showing only prefrontal distribution) and may be related to these volleys. It may have functional significance in the performance of this task and raises the possibility for this second hypothesis concerning the occurrence of prefrontal slow activity. This hypothesis is not necessarily restricted to the performance of sequential arithmetic problems because this activity could possibly occur in conjunction with interruptions during the performance of a mental task.

A third hypothesis relates the occurrence of anterior slow activity to the presence of FM theta [frontal midline theta, *Ishihara and Yoshii*, 1966; *Tani*, 1982]. They performed factor analyses of one bipolar derivation (F_z-C_z) for each of the traditional EEG frequency bands separately. These analyses were designed to study the degree of relationship that each of these frequency bands had with the administered tasks.

The main thrust was to determine the parameters governing the occurrence of frontal midline theta. They had previously established the presence of this activity while engaging in mental work, and subsequently they performed 2 sets of factor analyses, a factor analysis of the test scores administered and a set of factor analyses of the separate EEG frequency bands. Their main finding for the scalp area they studied (F_z-C_z) is that 2 factors evolve in the theta band, 1 which they identify as a thinking factor and another which seems to involve working speed.

With their design, however, it is not possible to determine the relationship that frequency bands have with each other nor, given the one derivation limitation, to obtain factors which furnish information about the interaction between the distribution of involved scalp areas and the distribution of EEG frequencies.

Figure 15/9 shows for the Resting I and II conditions factors loaded on the lower frequencies and localized primarily in the prefrontal areas. They are Resting I factor 9 and Resting II factor 5. While the first of the 2 factors accounts for 4% of the variance, Resting II factor 5 accounts for 6% of the variance. In addition, the latter has loadings in scattered areas and in particular in the parietal areas in faster frequencies. Noise factor 8 and Music factor 10 have distributions similar to the Resting I condition, but Voice factor 7 shows stronger loadings and additional loadings in the lateral frontal and temporal areas. Arithmetic factor 10 is the only factor in figure 15/9 showing strictly a prefrontal localization. It also has a broad frequency distribution of loadings.

The second and third hypotheses concerning prefrontal slow activity are not mutually exclusive. While the authors involved in FM-theta research interpreted this activity to be correlated with thinking activity, it may instead correlate with momentary pauses in the thinking activity and, as such, be intermixed in other conditions in which the investigators had not identified the thinking component. On the other hand, FM theta may be the anterior component of the portion of theta activity that in the present investigation was found to be positively related with the capacity for intellectual functions (cf. chapter 9 and *Liberson's* interpretation, chapter 13).

The patterning of prefrontal slow frequencies obtained shows clearly that this activity functions as a separate entity in a variety of biological states as evidenced in the 8 conditions studied (fig. 15/9). The present data does not permit a hierarchy of conditions regarding the relevance of this activity nor does it contain evidence to support the hypothesis concerning the role of FM theta in thinking, but it reaffirms the existence of this group of frequencies as constituting one or more separate entities in the prefrontal and anterior areas. The nature of this activity and its separation from possible contamination from eye-movement artifacts remain to be studied. It appears that, given the different distribution characteristics and the different frequency composition in the prefrontal areas, all of these factors cannot be postulated as deriving from a single cause, e.g. eye-movement artifacts.

Posterior Slow. By contrast, the posterior slow activity occurs only in 2 conditions, white Noise factor 2 (fig. 15/2) and mental Arithmetic factor 5 (fig. 15/5). The loadings are much stronger in Noise factor 2, and the distribution is broader probably as a consequence of the magnitude of the loading, but the strongest loadings are in the same areas for both conditions, namely occipital, parietal and post-temporal in a basically bilateral symmetrical pattern. The white Noise condition is a perceptually uncomfortable condition. Even though the noise level was not uncomfortably loud per se, the fact that the stimulation lacked figure provoked a figure-ground search in the brain. It is possible that this search for figure is expressed at least in part by this presence of slow activity in most posterior areas. Mental Arithmetic also involves a search for the appropriate response, and a possible parallel is thus available for the presence of a similar factor in these two conditions.

Prefrontal Fast. All but the 2 visual eyes-open conditions show a factor in this range. The distribution is almost completely in the prefrontal derivations except for Music where the factor includes 15-Hz activity in the central areas, for Voice where the factor includes 2-Hz activity primarily in posterior areas and in the Resting I and II conditions where this factor includes fast activity in the frontal areas as well. A portion of this activity may be due to forehead muscle artifacts, but it would be difficult to draw that conclusion in Music factor 7 (fig. 15/3) and Voice factor 8 (fig. 15/4) because of the broader distribution of the loadings throughout brain areas.

Anterior Fast. There is only 1 factor, Music factor 3 (fig. 15/3), which satisfies these characteristics in a primarily symmetrical distribution. The distribution includes frontal, central and primarily lateral frontal derivations, the frequency range being all the way from 13 to 33 Hz. The distribution shows an overall symmetry but with greater loadings in the left lateral frontal and in the right temporal areas in comparison with their homologous counterpart. Even though this is a unique distribution, it could be related to the 19- to 33-Hz activity discussed earlier and to the activity described under the right anterior, the right temporal and the lateral frontal headings as well as under the heading of left temporal fast to be discussed later. If this is the case, this cluster of factors would be sharing a basic mechanism for processing information in the brain.

Post-Temporal Fast. Another unique factor is the post-temporal fast factor which is found in factor 3 of the Resting II condition (fig. 15/8). No other condition shows this type of activity, not even the Resting I condition, underscoring the fact that the 2 Resting conditions are basically different, the first being one with greater unresolved tensions. This particular factor which is rather high in the hierarchy of factors in the Resting II condition may point to a particular role of the post-temporal derivations.

Occipital Fast. Three conditions, Resting I, white Noise and Diffuse vision, show a factor with loadings in the occipital fast range. This factor would point to the fact that both the white Noise and Diffuse vision conditions, even though under different perceptual modalities, are conditions without pattern. This absence of pattern may also be surmised to be present in the Resting I condition in which the subject, requested to lie still in a dark room with eyes closed, expects the unknown. This activity, therefore, could be related to a search for pattern and/or to an expression of expectation of unknown stimuli.

Right Anterior. This heading includes 2 different types of factors. The first type, Resting I factor 10 (not shown) and Noise factor 10 (not shown), involves the right frontal area in a frequency range from 19 to 25 Hz. These loadings are very small and account for a very small portion of the total variance. The other type of factor is the one shown by Voice factor 9 (fig. 15/4) and Resting II factor 8 (fig. 15/8) to be discussed in the next chapter together with the temporal factors.

Miscellaneous. Of the factors relegated to the miscellaneous category, there were factor 10 of 4 conditions as well as 3 other factors. These factors 10 are not displayed graphically and are described here.

Resting I factor 10 is characterized by 23-Hz loading in the left frontal area and 21- to 25-Hz loadings in the right frontal area. Noise factor 10 is characterized by 19- to 25-Hz loadings in the right frontal area. Voice factor 10 is characterized by 1-Hz loading in the left temporal and post-temporal as well as by 19-Hz loadings in the 2 frontal and right parietal areas. Diffuse vision factor 10 is characterized by one 25-Hz loading in the right central area. The 3 additional factors in this category, patterned vision factors 7 and 8 and Diffuse vision factor 9 are available in figures 15/6 and 15/7.

References

Frane, J.; Jennrich, R.: P4M: Factor analysis; in Dixon, Brown, BMDP-79, Biomedical Computer Programs, P-Series, pp. 656–684 (University of California Press, Berkeley 1979).

Giannitrapani, D.: Sex differences in EEG spectra. Electroenceph. clin. Neurophysiol. *37:* 434–435 (1974).

Giannitrapani, D.: Laterality preference, electrophysiology and the brain. Electromyogr. clin. Neurophysiol. *19:* 105–123 (1979a).

Giannitrapani, D.: EEG correlates of sex and schizophrenia. Soc. Neurosci. Abstr., p. 205 (Nov., 1979b).

Giannitrapani, D.: Sex differences in the electrophysiology of the higher cortical functions. Electroenceph. clin. Neurophysiol. *52:* S136 (1981).

Giannitrapani, D.: Distribution of EEG power and coherence relating to gender. Neuroscience *7:* suppl., p. S80 (1982).

Giannitrapani, D.; Kayton, L.: Schizophrenia and EEG spectral analysis. Electroenceph. clin. Neurophysiol. *36:* 377–386 (1974).

Harman, H.H.: Modern factor analysis; 2nd ed. (University of Chicago Press, Chicago 1967).

Ishihara, T.; Yoshii, N.: Activation of abnormal EEG by mental work (in Japanese). Rinsho Noha/Clin. Electroenceph. *8:* 26–34 (1966).

Jennrich, R.I.; Sampson, P.F.: Rotation for simple loadings. Psychometrika *31:* 313–323 (1966).

Löwenhard, P.: P factor analysis of single EEG recordings. Göteborg psychol. Rep. *3:* 1–14 (1973).

Tani, K.: Psychological factors of frontal midline theta waves – changes by repeated mental tasks. Bull. Osaka Pref. Coll. Nurs. *4:* 117–122 (1982).

16 Interaction between Left and Right Temporal Regions

> Ideas, to become thought, are captured by the brain which bounces
> them to and fro in a continuous attempt to place them into a structure
> that never enclosed them before.
> *Duilio Giannitrapani*

The factors dealing with the anterior lateral areas are being discussed separately because of the relevance they have in the processing of higher cortical functions. Factors loaded on these areas have been rearranged in figures 16/1 and 16/2. It can be shown at a glance that these factors have a distribution of loadings which is at times symmetrical and at times homologously asymmetrical. For the sake of consistency, discussion will first conclude the analysis of table 15/I after which a general discussion of the multifaceted activity of the temporal areas will follow.

Right Anterior

Voice factor 9 and Resting II factor 8 show a distribution primarily right lateral frontal, and the frequency range is in a broad range from 5 to 33 Hz. In addition, Voice factor 9 shows loadings in the frontal and central areas in the 31-Hz activity. If one combines Voice factor 2 and Voice factor 9 the resulting pattern is reminiscent of the pattern shown in the next category which has, however, a primarily right temporal and lateral frontal distribution.

Right Temporal and Lateral Frontal

This is a very important factor which includes the first factor under the Noise, the Arithmetic and the Diffuse vision conditions. Noise and Diffuse vision are the 2 conditions without pattern, 1 auditory and 1 visual, while Arithmetic is the only condition which requires a search for an internal pattern, the sine qua non for the performance of mental arithmetic. The distribution is anterior, includes fast activity and is somewhat asymmetrical with greater loadings in the right temporal and lateral frontal derivations.

Left Temporal Fast

In contrast with the preceding category, the left temporal fast (Voice factor 2) is the best expression of the asymmetry of the Voice condition with a traditional asymmetry of processing of verbal material in the lateral frontal and temporal areas. This factor is also present in the 2 Resting conditions and in the Music condition. Taking the Music condition first, Music factor 9 shows weak loadings in the left temporal at frequencies from 19 to 33 Hz and does not show the lateral frontal component present in Voice factor 2.

In the Resting I condition, instead, there is a large lateral frontal component and a broad distribution of loadings in the 1-Hz band. In the Resting II condition the loadings are very weak and restricted to lateral frontal frequency in the 27-Hz and temporal frequency in the 15- and 23- to 27-Hz bands. These 2 resting factors can be interpreted as indicating the presence of internal speech in the 2 Resting conditions with a decrease of this activity in the Resting II condition.

What conclusion can be drawn from the pattern of distributions of frequency loadings in the left and right temporal regions? Inspection of figure 16/2 shows that Vision factor 1 has the greatest number of strong loadings distributed throughout brain areas with somewhat greater loadings in the left of the lateral frontal areas. Diffuse vision shows somewhat similar but weaker loadings with a major difference, i.e. the asymmetry in this case consists of stronger loadings in the right temporal area. The basic difference between the 2 conditions is that in the latter the visual stimulation has no pattern.

There is one other condition in which stimulation has no pattern, i.e. listening to white Noise, and factor 1 of this condition (fig. 15/2 and 16/1) shows a similar pattern to that of Diffuse vision factor 1. The similarity of the 2 conditions points to a particular role of the right temporal area for processing stimuli that do not have a structure.

Inspection of all the factors having temporal loadings (fig. 16/1 and 16/2) shows that stronger loadings on the right of the 2 temporal regions occur also in factor 1 of the Arithmetic condition. In this condition, the subject is required to perform mentally sequential subtractions, i.e. to find an internal structure which permits resolution of the problem. Arguing back from the presently available data, one could conclude that an asymmetry of temporal activity with greater loadings on the right side is a correlate of a search for structure, be it internal or external.

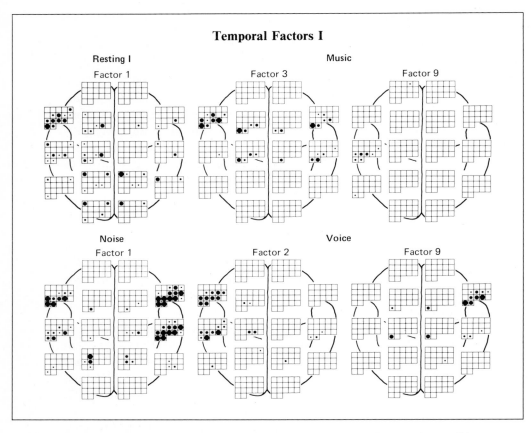

Fig. 16/1. The temporal factors for the Resting I, Noise, Music and Voice conditions, shown separately with the other factors of each analysis in figures 15/1–15/8, are regrouped to facilitate comparison.

Additional information of the role of the lateralization of temporal activity is given by the Voice condition which shows a separation of the activity of the 2 temporal lobes into 2 factors: Voice factor 2 with clear left lateral frontal and temporal loadings which seem to satisfy the traditional expectation of speech localization in those areas and Voice factor 9 which shows the other half of the distribution in the right lateral frontal and temporal areas. The variances are different, with Voice factor 2 accounting for 9% of the variance while Voice factor 9 accounts for only 5% of the variance.

Music also shows a separation of the temporal activity into 2 factors, Music factor 3 (fig. 16/1), primarily bilateral but with almost no loading on the left temporal area, while Music factor 9 concentrates on the left tempo-

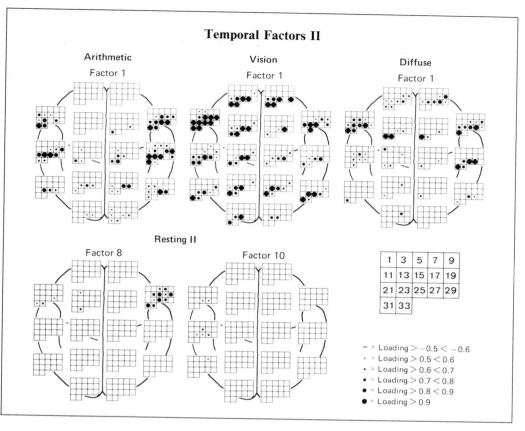

Fig. 16/2. The temporal factors for the Arithmetic, patterned Vision, Diffuse vision and Resting II conditions, shown separately with the other factors of each analysis in figures 15/1–15/8, are regrouped to facilitate comparison.

ral area. Additional research is needed to develop an understanding of the mechanisms involved in processing musical stimuli. It is sufficient to state at this time that the separation in the Music and the Voice conditions of the temporal activity into 2 factors may constitute an item of particular significance for those functions.

The 2 Resting conditions also show differences. Resting I (fig. 16/1) is primarily loaded on the left side with additional scattered posterior loadings. It could be an indication that during this condition the subject was not really at rest but perhaps was repeating to himself the last instructions which were given to him since the loadings are reminiscent of those in Voice factor 2. By contrast, Resting II (fig. 16/2) divides this activity into 2 factors, factor 8 primarily loaded in the right lateral frontal area and factor 10 primarily loaded in the left temporal area. Note the absence of loadings in the right temporal area, characteristic of Arithmetic factor 1, Noise factor 1 and Diffuse vision factor 1, indicating that this resting condition is indeed processing something different from those conditions.

On the left side a different pattern occurred. In Resting II factor 10 the loadings are primarily temporal, a situation which occurred also in Music factor 9. Without presuming to have covered the complex role that the temporal and lateral frontal areas serve in the processing of higher cortical functions, there is enough differentiation in the 8 conditions given to indicate certain roles for these areas. It should be emphasized at this point that the correlational studies of chapter 9 dealt with data that was basically unrelated to the task in question. Those correlational studies did include data based on an average of the 8 conditions, and for any significant correlations to occur, a specific condition could contribute only one eighth of the variance. In chapters 15 and 16, however, the data was obtained during the performance of the specific tasks. In chapter 9, the data referring to temporal and lateral frontal areas and dealing with the relationship between EEG power and intellectual functions show different patterns of lateralization depending on the subtest involved. Rather than interpreting those relationships in light of the factor analysis findings, this investigator leaves that task to the reader in the expectation of generating more research in this area.

In conclusion, the patterns observed indicate that the different conditions include separate functions that can be studied experimentally with electrophysiological methods. It can also be concluded that even though the Voice condition has a factor which is asymmetrically loaded on the left side, the fact that this asymmetry is found only in 1 of the factors indicates that the processing of voice is performed by involving the whole brain and concerns several very specific functions even in the right lateral frontal area of the brain as shown in Voice factor 9.

The arithmetic functions, by contrast, have been variously attributed to occupying the left side because of its verbal component and the right side because of the findings with patients with acalculia. The clinical findings, however, have never been experimentally clear because of the involvement of other brain areas, and this factor analysis of the mental Arithmetic condition seems to clearly separate the components of factor 1 which involves the bilateral brain areas primarily on the right side, factor 3 which involves central areas, factor 2 which involves central posterior areas and factor 4 which involves prefrontal areas.

V Epilogue

'It seems to me that the human race stands on the brink of a major breakthrough. We have advanced to the point where we can put our hand on the hem of the curtain that separates us from an understanding of the nature of our minds. Is it conceivable that we will withdraw our hand and turn back through discouragement and lack of vision?'
P.W. Bridgman

17 Neurophysiological Considerations and the Scanning Theory

'We must not expect one blinding flash of discovery. Instead we have to dare to put up hypotheses that attempt partial explanations ...'
Sir *John Eccles*

The following interpretation of the possible neural mechanisms involved in the execution of higher cortical functions is based on *Eccles'* [1951] formulation. He maintained that frequency of alpha activity at around 10 Hz is readily explained if it is due to circulation of impulses in closed self-reexciting chains. After the discharge of an impulse, recovery from depressed excitability is almost complete by 100 ms, and when a neural network is subjected to continuous bombardment of low intensity, such as when cortical activity is at a low level, the probability of a subsequent discharge will reach a maximum at about 100 ms. In a network of closed self-reexciting chains with a low level of cortical activity, therefore, frequencies in the alpha range would be those most likely generated.

It would also follow that with a higher cortical excitation level, a higher level of bombardment of the neuron at the synaptic junction would occur with the result that the neuron would be excited in a shorter period than the above-mentioned 100 ms. The minimum lag would be approximately 15 ms, the absolute refractory period during which a stimulus of any strength is incapable of generating a neuronal response. The theoretical upper limit of the frequency generated by closed self-reexciting chains would therefore be 66 Hz. This does not preclude the existence in the EEG of frequencies higher than 66 Hz which could be the resultant of either the interaction of several of these circuits or of different methods of generation. Higher frequencies have been observed, for instance, by *Bremer* [1944], *Spillberg* [1947] and *Trabka* [1962].

Some of these chains can be postulated to perform a scanning function. Historically, the scanning construct has been almost exclusively relegated to alpha activity. *Pitts and McCulloch* [1947] developed a model to account for the scanning of afferent visual and auditory processes. They related the phase differences of alpha activity in different cerebral structures to the processing of these afferents. Their ideas were further elaborated by *McCulloch* [1951], who demonstrated a relationship between the frequency of alpha activity and the frequency at which musical chords or visual forms can be distinguished.

Walter [1950] also spoke of the alpha activity of the EEG as a scanning mechanism and postulated the existence of other scanning mechanisms. He discussed specifically the appearance of theta activity in conjunction with pleasure withdrawal and indicated that this slow potential may represent scanning for pleasure.

Beta activity, because of its small amplitude, was not studied in this context before *Mundy-Castle's* [1951] work. He concluded that a portion of beta activity, appearing at the inception of the stimulus and disappearing soon after, could represent scansion of cortical projection and association areas.

The plausibility of such scanning hypotheses in EEG is therefore supported by the disappearance of EEG activities in conjunction with the introduction of new stimulation in some cases or with an increase in specificity of stimulation in others [*Giannitrapani,* 1971]. The predictability or higher regularity of a circuit would be expressed in the EEG with higher voltage in a narrower frequency band. The correlations between intellectual performance and power might be simply a measure of the regularity with which these neural circuits are available to the working mind.

What we might be observing in the matrices of correlations between intellectual tasks and EEG is the activity produced in a myriad of such self-reexciting chains. Since the EEGs used are unrelated to the intellectual task in question, it can be postulated that the strength of these circuits is related to their availability for performing an intellectual task in proportion to their regularity which permits better synchronization between neuronal chains and therefore more predictable, more efficient and faster transfer of information. Support for this notion can be observed in correlations of the slow beta frequencies of the EEG taken during the Arithmetic condition (table 9/XV) and more generally can be sought in table 7/I. Each one of these frequencies may be the resultant of one or more such chains.

It is not presumed here that the electrophysiological complexity of the performance of an intellectual task is fully comprehended nor that the most significant circuits involved have been detected. These may number in the hundreds for even the most simple intellectual task.

Setting aside the neurophysiological model, *Giannitrapani* [1971] had been able to observe in the raw EEG spectra changes in the distribution of fast beta activity (20–34 Hz) which were related to the different conditions of stimulation during EEG recording. The distribution of these EEG beta activity changes was such that this beta activity could be hypothesized to constitute an internal scanning for structure as contrasted to an external scanning served by alpha activity. The following rationale for a hierarchy of scanning mechanisms was developed.

Alpha activity can be thought of as scanning for any stimulation; its function ceases or subsides in the presence of a broad range of percepts whether internal or external. At this point in the perceptual cycle, faster scanning mechanisms come into play as exemplified by high beta activity in the temporal areas (scanning for structure). This activity is governed by the same laws governing alpha activity, and it subsides when the conditions for its existence are no longer present, i.e. when the stimulus has acquired structure. Beta activity was found to increase in the temporal areas for all of the 8 conditions used but was also observed in the occipital areas in the Diffuse vision condition and in the prefrontal areas for the white Noise, Voice and Arithmetic conditions, all conditions in which a continuous search for structure can be postulated.

The postulation of the existence of a scanning activity in the performance of higher cortical functions is supported by the work of *Sternberg* [1966] who was able to isolate two such scanning processes relating to the retrieval of short-term memory. His work will be briefly described here because it constitutes supporting evidence for scanning activity in a field unrelated to EEG phenomena.

Sternberg [1966] gave subjects series of digits of different length to memorize. When the subject was presented with a test digit he was to press a button to indicate whether that digit was included in the original series. The length of time required for a response was linear with the increase of the number of digits in the memorized series at a speed of 20–30 digits/s. *Sternberg* called this an internal serial-comparison process, and it coincides with the frequencies of high beta activity postulated by *Giannitrapani* [1971] to consist of an internal scanning for structure. Both investigators may be over- or under-inclusive in their definition because of their narrow experimental approach to the phenomenon, but the importance of *Sternberg's* finding is the linearity in the increments of time required for processing with the increase in the length of the series, a finding which makes a strong case for a single processing function for that activity.

Sternberg's case has been corroborated and expanded by *Koh* et al. [1977] in their work with schizophrenic processing of verbal material. They were able to conclude that in schizophrenics short-term memory was intact and that their slowness in response was to be understood in terms of some dysfunction in their stimulus encoding response selection and/or response execution.

Subsequent work of *Sternberg* [1967] demonstrated another linear function for the retrieval, from a short recently memorized list, of the digit that follows a test digit. In this paradigm in which the task is more complex than a simple recognition, the processing speed has an average rate of 4 digits/s, suggesting the existence of a much slower scanning mechanism.

One should not conclude from the foregoing that a couple of scanning frequencies might be sufficient to process perceptual phenomena. The complexity of the situation was summarized by *Cavanagh* [1972] who was able to compile another linear function for a full memory search corresponding to a frequency of 4/s. *Cavanagh* began by compiling a number of studies dealing with different classes of stimuli (digits, colors, letters, words, geometrical shapes, random forms and nonsense syllables). Each class of stimuli had a characteristic reaction time. However, when multiplying the reaction time for a single item times the maximum number of items for a given class, he found a constant of 243.2 ms. This indicated that each class of items was scanned at a different speed but that scanning of the full memory was always executed at a speed of 4/s. One can only conclude that the capacity of the full memory is a constant and that the number of items that can be stored depends on the complexity of each item, but this also means that different scanning frequencies are available for items of different degrees of complexity. These findings were obtained from mean data, and therefore individual variations need to be studied.

One, however, can postulate the existence of a hierarchy of scanning mechanisms, consisting at one level of frequencies responsible for search of individual items and at another level of 4/s activity at which point these items have already obtained a certain level of organization and become available for further processing. In EEG this latter mechanism belongs to the group of frequencies known as theta activity of which very little is known except that it acquires dominance in drowsiness and in conditions in which cortical control is poor. In a field unrelated to EEG, frequencies in the 4/s range are evident in conjunction with damage to motor functions as in the case of Parkinsonian tremor. This negative valence of 4/s activity is

counteracted by the work of *Sternberg* and *Cavanagh* who identified functions served in this frequency range, as mentioned above.

Furthermore, the evidence in the present study (cf. the data presented
in chapter 9) indicated a positive relationship between the level of performance for certain verbal subtests and EEG theta activity (3–7 Hz). This
may be due to the presence of theta activity components facilitating the
performance of certain mental functions such as the one described above.

In addition, it is particularly rewarding that *Giannitrapani's* [1971]
detailed description of scanning functions is supported by the factor analysis findings of a separate sample as can be observed in the patterning of the
factors in chapters 15 and 16. This analysis also corroborated the asymmetry of the internal search for structure observed earlier by *Giannitrapani*
[1971]. More specifically the temporal asymmetry in the power of these fast
beta frequencies (with greater power on the right side) was reflected in the
factor analyses with greater loadings on the right side for these frequencies
in those areas. This relationship between power and loadings is not to be
interpreted as that the loadings are proportional to power but rather that a
greater portion of the power of the fast beta activity in the right temporal
area is involved in the function subsumed by the factor in question. A
dominant role in this internal search for structure by the right temporal area
seems to be thus clearly established.

In an attempt to place this scanning hypothesis in the broader framework of information-processing mechanisms of the brain, support for these
mechanisms will be sought in the perceptual domain. If this scanning
hypothesis is correct, it would be reasonable to expect that such mechanisms would govern perceptual as well as conceptual functions.

Support for this hypothesis is found, e.g. in the evidence that reaction
time varies with the phase of the alpha cycle [*Lansing,* 1957]. This excitability cycle was also found to relate to the latencies of the evoked potentials
[*Dustman and Beck,* 1965]. In light of this point of contact between reaction
time and the evoked potentials, the investigations attempting to establish a
relationship between evoked potentials and intellectual functions can be
viewed as studying a particular aspect of the reaction-time paradigm.

In addition to reaction time, another readily available measure in perception is critical flicker frequency. Early intelligence investigations attempted correlations with both measures with the hypothesis that faster
reaction time and a higher critical flicker fusion are a measure of speed of
performance, hence perhaps a measure of a critical factor in intellectual
functioning. *Halstead* [1947] found low positive correlations, and *Tanner*

[1950], manipulating the dark period of the CFF, found correlations as high as 0.5 with language scores while *Crovitz* et al. [1971] found the limit for imaging flicker of about 4/s.

The fact, however, that these experiments indicated that reaction times and CFFs were influenced by a variety of parameters such as duration interval, intensity and size of the stimulus led to the conclusion that the measurement obtained constituted a sample of the neurophysiological makeup of the individual in a very restricted sense, meaningful only in the context of many qualifiers. The matter is further complicated by the inter-action of stimulus duration and luminance as studied by *Raab and Fehrer* [1962].

Within the framework of the neural model derived from *Eccles* [1951], the failure of the perceptual literature to yield findings on specific frequen-cies can be explained. One of the early laws established in perception research is Ricco's law which specifies an equivalency between brightness and area of given visual stimulus. To explain the phenomenon, a summa-tion of networks was adduced, not unlike the mechanism adduced by the neurophysiological model under consideration.

There is one fundamental difference, however, between the require-ments of perceptual and conceptual circuits. In perception, summation serves a fundamental role in dealing with the size/intensity dimension in order to translate it into a signal of stimulus strength, stimulus closeness or imminence of an impending stimulus. In the conceptual sphere these parameters are secondary to coding of language parameters whose salient feature is the number and speed with which this coding can take place rather than perceptual magnitude. Neural summation then in this model of con-ceptual phenomena is relinquished from the role it serves in perception and would serve perhaps a lesser role. If this is true, scanning frequencies in the model for conception would be easier to identify because of their being less subject to fluctuations due to summation and its role in perception.

References

Bremer, F.: L'activité 'spontanée' des centres nerveux. Bull. Acad. méd. Belg. *11:* 148–173 (1944).

Cavanagh, J.P.: Relation between the immediate memory span and the memory search rate. Psychol. Rev. *79:* 525–530 (1972).

Crovitz, H.F.; Rosof, D.; Schiffman, H.: Timing oscillation in human visual imagery. Psychon. Sci. *24:* 87–88 (1971).

Dustman, R.E.; Beck, E.C.: Phase of alpha brain waves, reaction time and visually evoked potentials. Electroenceph. clin. Neurophysiol. *18:* 433–440 (1965).

Eccles, J.C.: Interpretation of action potentials evoked in the cerebral cortex. Electroenceph. clin. Neurophysiol. *3:* 449–464 (1951).

Giannitrapani, D.: Scanning mechanisms and the EEG. Electroenceph. clin. Neurophysiol. *30:* 139–146 (1971).

Halstead, W.C.: Brain and intelligence, a quantitative study of the frontal lobes (University of Chicago Press, Chicago 1947).

Koh, S.D.; Szoc, R.; Peterson, R.A.: Short-term memory scanning in schizophrenic young adults. J. abnorm. soc. Psychol. *86:* 451–460 (1977).

Lansing, R.W.: Relation of brain and tremor rhythms to visual reaction time. Electroenceph. clin. Neurophysiol. *9:* 497–504 (1957).

McCulloch, W.S.: Why the mind is in the head; in Jeffress, Cerebral mechanisms in behavior. The Hixon Symp., pp. 72–141 (Wiley, New York 1951).

Mundy-Castle, A.C.: Theta and beta rhythm in the electroencephalograms of normal adults. Electroenceph. clin. Neurophysiol. *3:* 477–486 (1951).

Pitts, W.; McCulloch, W.S.: How we know universals: the perception of auditory and visual forms. Bull. math. Biophys. *9:* 127–147 (1947).

Raab, D.; Fehrer, E.: Supplementary report: the effect of stimulus duration and luminance on visual reaction time. J. exp. Psychol. *64:* 326–327 (1962).

Spillberg, P.I.: Quick potentials of the human brain and their significance in the normal and in pathology. Biulletin Eksperimental Noi Biologgi I Meditsiny *23:* 124–128 (1947).

Sternberg, S.: High speed scanning in human memory. Science *153:* 652–654 (1966).

Sternberg, S.: Retrieval of contextual information from memory. Psychon. Sci. *8:* 55–56 (1967).

Tanner, W.P., Jr.: A preliminary investigation of the relationship between visual fusion of intermittent light and intelligence. Science *112:* 201–203 (1950).

Trabka, J.: High frequency components in brain wave activity. Electroenceph. clin. Neurophysiol. *14:* 453–464 (1962).

Walter, W.G.: The twenty-fourth Maudsley lecture: the functions of the electrical rhythms in the brain. J. ment. Sci. *96:* 1–31 (1950).

18 Conclusions

'Inventions are accepted not when they are invented but when the world can no longer do without them.'
Buckminster Fuller

(1) The existence of frequency components of steady-state EEG that are related to higher cortical functions has been amply demonstrated.

(2) Within this overall finding, specific frequency components that relate to the capacity for aspects of mental activity have been isolated.

(3) The differential involvement of brain areas, as measured at the scalp, relating to the capacity for different types of mental activity has also been demonstrated.

(4) Corroborating these findings are the findings concerning the frequency changes in EEG activity during the performance of mental activity. The changes occurred in frequency bands (15 and 17 Hz) identical to those which correlated with mental Arithmetic in the steady-state EEG.

(5) 13-Hz activity, and in particular its presence in central areas, was shown to be pivotal as a correlate of the capacity for mentation as studied in the present investigation.

(6) Studies of mental ability obtained from the literature employing factor analysis of the Wechsler Intelligence Scale for Children (WISC) permitted the conclusion that 13-Hz activity is involved in the performance of verbal functions as observed in the early analysis of the data showing a relationship between 13-Hz activity and verbal subtests.

(7) Factor analysis of the EEG under different behavioral states was demonstrated to be a useful and powerful method in the study of the localization of higher cortical functions.

(8) In the execution of higher cortical functions the overall activity was shown to be overwhelmingly homologously symmetrical even among those functions for which asymmetries had been noted in the literature, asymmetries which had been magnified as representing the overwhelming characteristics of those functions.

(9) Besides the observation of the lateralization of Broca's areas for speech on the left side, the right temporal areas were shown to have an important role which can be described as one of searching for perceptual organization.

(10) The relationships between EEG and mental activity were found to be slightly higher in general on the left side of the brain even among left-handers. This may be due to the fact that when comparing homologous brain areas the EEG on the left side is more reliable. This reliability differential needs to be studied because it may be close to the source of the cause of brain dominance.

(11) Numerous additional points concerning the relationship between the presence of EEG frequency components in specific locations and their relationships with higher cortical functions or clinical findings have been made throughout the book. The majority of such occurrences have been left uninterpreted. Further interpretation is left to the readers and their clinical knowledge or experience in the field of mental abilities.

Corroboration of EEG-Mentation Frequency Correlates

The relationship between Verbal IQ and 13-Hz activity in most of 16 brain areas surfaced time and again in several analyses of this study and was found to be very resilient. It was strongest in the central areas. This particular concentration was somewhat difficult to interpret because the current body of neuropsychological knowledge does not include an established intellectual role for these areas.

There is a known poor correlation between skull landmarks and underlying cortical structures. When the scalp locations are derived by subdividing the distances between points on the scalp, the variation with cortical structures is even greater. On the average, however, the central electrode placements can be thought of as corresponding to an area anterior to the precentral gyrus (the latter presiding over motor functions), i.e. the pre-motor area which is vaguely associated with motor functions. *Luria* [1966] ascribed to this area a more specific intellectual function, having observed lesions of this area as being related to intellectual deficits concerned with the inability to synthesize and automate mental activity.

The central placements of the present study are the closest ones to the supplementary motor areas on the medial surface between the two hemispheres [*Penfield and Roberts,* 1969]. These areas when cortically stimulated produced vague movements and unintelligible speech articulations and seemed to offer no specific interest. *Eccles and Robinson* [1984] concluded that, since impulses appear in the supplementary motor area prior to the initiation of movement and ostensibly prior to the appearance of impulses anywhere else in the brain, the supplementary motor area is the closest neurophysiological evidence of mind.

In the context of 13-Hz activity, *Weinberg* [1969], interested in studying alpha activity and using spectral analysis of visual evoked potentials, investigated the 2 occipital areas in which alpha activity is primarily present. He obtained a positive correlation between Verbal IQ and amplitude of 12- to 14-Hz components of visual evoked potentials.

It is difficult to conceptualize physiologically *Weinberg's* finding as well as other findings of spectral analysis of evoked potentials because the spectral analysis methodology requires the removal of the data from the time domain while evoked potential data is event-related. When inspected in its original time domain form, evoked potential data has characteristics which are different for each subsequent segment of time. In contrast, the spectral analysis of steady-state EEG can assume that each subsequent time segment has equal valence. This assumption can be made both on theoretical and empirical grounds, in the first case because steady-state EEG is not event-related, i.e. does not occur in time after a triggering stimulus, and in the second case because visual inspection can conclude that a subsequent EEG segment has features that could have occurred in a preceding segment or vice versa. This justifies obtaining an integral value for the frequencies occurring during an EEG time segment. An integral value of frequency components from an evoked potential time segment is more difficult to justify. Be that as it may, after finding the presence of frequency components in the spectral analysis of evoked potentials, finding a correlation between the amplitude of this frequency component and Verbal IQ is difficult to understand.

Osaka and Osaka's [1980] research supported *Weinberg's* finding. They observed with a monopolar occipital electrode in the midline a 12-Hz peak in the spectral analysis of visual evoked potentials in normal subjects, while in mentally retarded subjects this peak was absent.

The extensive information on 13-Hz activity developed in the present study indicates that 13-Hz activity is not an isolated evoked potential finding. In an attempt to coordinate *Weinberg's* and *Osaka and Osaka's* findings with those of the present study, it could be hypothesized that their 13-Hz component consists also of an EEG steady-state component. The following 2 conditions must be present: (1) It would be necessary that the 13-Hz component have a phase which resets itself in synchrony with the stimulus used for triggering the evoked potential, and (2) this 13-Hz component would also need to be phase-locked in time. Both conditions are necessary for a steady-state component to survive averaging, the latter being a sine qua non of the evoked potential methodology. Whether this interpretation represents the actual state of affairs remains to be investigated.

While *Weinberg's* and *Osaka and Osaka's* findings suggest the presence in the upper range of the alpha band of a frequency component related to either Verbal IQ or Full-Scale IQ, in light of the findings of the present study restricting investigations to 1 or 2 brain areas does not justify the implicit assumption that the presence of frequencies in those brain areas is representative of the brain as a whole. The present study demonstrated that occipital areas are the least involved in the relationship between 13-Hz activity and verbal functioning. Furthermore, the significance of their relationships is not particularly strong among the areas traditionally known to be involved in verbal or speech functions.

The findings of the present research were not restricted to 13-Hz activity. Both slower and faster activity were found to have their own specific patterns of relationships with mental functions. In regard to slower activity such as, for instance, the one found to relate in a broad range of brain areas to WISC Comprehension, it might be relevant to point out that some observations have already been made in animals concerning the presence of 4- to 6-Hz activity in the hippocampus and mental functions. *Adey* [1969], for instance, both with traditional EEG, spectral analysis of the EEG and spectral analysis of evoked potentials found in the hippocampus of the cat a complex pattern of relationships between 4- and 6-Hz activity during alerting, orienting and discriminative behavior. The significance of slow activity in the context of higher cortical functions was discussed in chapter 9 and, more specifically, it is central to *Liberson's* (chapter 13) interpretation of these data.

Maturation Issue

EEG variables historically related to intellectual functions were maturational in nature. The majority of the parameters studied consisted of various measures of occipital alpha often related to mental retardation. A developmental hypothesis was either expressed or implied, and even the latest more sophisticated attempt [*Gasser* et al., 1983] consisted of broad frequency band parameters which yielded stronger relationships with intellectual variables in the mentally defective sample as compared with a normal sample. The strategy adopted by that study predicted stronger correlations in specific diagnostic groups rather than in the population at large. Since correlation theory predicts stronger correlations in a population reflecting a broader range of the variable in question, the prediction of *Gasser* et al. [1983] implies that the stronger correlations they found in the narrowly defined pathological groups is due to variance of the parameters from within the pathology in question. In their case, working with a mentally defective group, both the theory of mental retardation, which specifies a slowing in intellectual growth, and the known developmental progression of EEG frequencies, which specifies an increase in the speed of EEG frequencies with age prior to adulthood, made the developmental interpretation of the inverse relationship between EEG and IQ reasonable and tenable.

The unique feature of the present study is that certain components of EEG activity within each frequency band are positively related to mental activity while other components of the same frequency band are negatively related to age. A reasonable, even if not necessary, conclusion is that these 2 sets of components are distinct and contribute separately and orthogonally to the total variance introduced by the power of a given EEG frequency. It is for this reason that the restriction suggested by *Gasser* et al. [1983] and *John* et al. [1980] in their neurometric studies, i.e. standardization of norms for given population subgroups, is not as necessary for the variables studied in the present investigation.

The presence of EEG frequency components positively related to mental abilities (in the present study) and the presence in the same frequency bands of a portion of the maturational components inversely related to mental abilities (in other studies), however, poses a problem for the emergence of findings in the present study. The result is one of masking the findings of the present study to the extent that these inversely related components are present. Some kind of age standardization of EEG parameters, similar perhaps to the one used by *John* et al. [1980], would increase the magnitude of the correlations obtained in this study.

The fact that the EEG frequency components related to mental functions was not related to age in this study contributes to the strength of the present data in many ways. First is the above-mentioned fact that this data is orthogonal to maturation which is positively related to age. Second and more important is the fact that, given this lack of relationship with maturation, these data are meaningful in a broad spectrum of the population without having to take into consideration maturational variables.

It should be emphasized at this point that the fact that the EEG parameters which are found to relate positively to mental functions and negatively to age does not necessarily mean that the frequency components responsible for the positive relationship between EEG and mental functions are negatively related to age. They are most probably orthogonal to age. The fact that a given EEG frequency band does not represent a unitary function is not new in EEG, and the work of *Katada* et al. [1981] is the latest example of an effort to demonstrate the topographic and maturational diversity of dominant frequencies both cross-sectionally and longitudinally.

The puzzle still remains as to why the frequency components which relate to mental functions in this study have not been observed before. The answer possibly lies in the fact that maturational components were more easily observable in the early work [*Knott* et al., 1942; *Liberson,* 1950] by visual inspection. After this early work frustrations over the relatively low correlations obtained and theoretical limitations furnished by these findings which indicated that the EEG at best could only furnish a measure representing a maturational correlate produced a vacuum in the search for physiological correlates of mental functions, a vacuum which was broken by *Giannitrapani* [1969, 1970, 1973] and now by *Gasser* et al. [1983].

A possible technical reason for the lack of these EEG-mental function findings not maturationally related is the fact that these findings have a very specific topographic and frequency distribution which were maximized in the present investigation by studies of the distribution of activity in 16 frequency bands across 16 brain areas. The work of *Gasser* et al. [1983], for instance, relied upon 6 broad frequency bands and 8 brain areas. While the latter may be adequate for EEG maturational analysis, the difference between the 2 studies is in the availability of 48 variables in the latter against 256 in the former, a figure which still could be profitably increased to obtain a better topographic and frequency definition of parameters.

Factor Analysis of the Wechsler Tests

In the search for the components of the *general* factor in intelligence, a major shortcoming of the traditional application of the factor analysis methodology is the fact that the question cannot be addressed in the abstract. The resultant loadings relate to the commonality of the variables explored. The choice of variables, therefore, is the determinant of what is being found as being common to those variables.

The application of the factor analysis technique adopted in this study obviates that shortcoming and permits the observation of truly new data. It is true that the loading is still dependent upon the choice of intellectual variables, but the factor loadings do not constitute the end product as in the traditional application of factor analysis. In this investigation they constitute the raw data that, once compared with EEG variables, permit the generation of new information having electrophysiological relevance. The power of this technique is that it makes possible the comparison of factors obtained in different studies with different rotations to demonstrate the degree of relationship that these factors have among themselves and to brain activity. The most arbitrary step in the factor analysis methodology is at what point the rotation of the factors is terminated for purposes of display, communication and discussion; hence the caution against inferring real clusters from a particular point in the rotation, i.e. a certain set of loadings whose grouping is an artifact of the point of rotation in question.

The application adopted in the present study permits a comparison of seemingly unrelated factors or factors having different clusters in the distribution of their loadings with an outside criterion, EEG variables. The data demonstrated that practically identical distribution of EEG activity was obtained with a variety of factors having seemingly unrelated loadings both in the same and different factor analyses. At this point then, it is correct to speak of electrophysiological clusters of activity.

To recapitulate the findings, there is ample evidence for 13-Hz activity to be related to the capacity for verbal functioning. There is also the confirmation that faster (low beta) activity is a component of EEG activity related to the capacity for numerical functioning and the confirmation that occipital activity, and in particular left occipital, is related to Performance IQ. The asymmetry of this finding is emphasized by the fact that these higher correlations of the left side survive the observed lower reliability of the EEG signal on the left of the 2 occipital areas as shown in figure 3/5.

The 23-Hz activity cluster, again related to verbal functioning, is also to be noted. It has come to the fore partially because of the extraordinarily high reliability of the signal (fig. 3/5). This area is inviting research both as to the nature of the 23-Hz activity to explain the reason for its reliability and to the function of this activity for the determination of whether it is related to a peripheral or central component of verbal functioning.

Wechsler's life-long wish [personal communication, Annual Meeting of the American Psychological Association, Miami 1970] was to be able to demonstrate physiological correlates to intellectual functions. He was poignantly aware that it was not possible to identify or equate general intelligence with intellectual ability, however defined [*Wechsler,* 1949], and took the novel position that an intelligence test measured something more rather than less than sheer intellectual ability. He described the vain attempts of using statistical procedures employed to reduce the contribution of factors such as traits (e.g. persistence, drive, energy level, etc.), vain because the net effect was often to diminish rather than to increase the validity of the tests as effective measures of general intelligence. He did not regard general intelligence as a unitary trait or ability. To the contrary, he postulated that intellectual capacity may be. While it is not in the scope of this study to determine the validity of these assertions, it is relevant to note that *Wechsler* did not conceptualize intelligence as a two-tiered structure (capacity versus current functioning). He subdivided the capacity component into an intrinsic ability, perhaps Spearman g, and surrounding traits heretofore not easily separable from the former which he referred to as general intelligence (not to be confused with g).

In light of the findings of the present investigation, it must be argued further that in the process of getting closer to the study of g it will probably become apparent that g itself is not a unitary function but that it can be subdivided into several components. The components referred to are not those being proposed by alternate factor-analytic investigators arguing whether g can be separated into several underlying traits. The components referred to are physiological components such as EEG frequency parameters which combine in a unique admixture in every individual to permit a unique capacity for performance that at a nonphysiological level results in an inseparable g factor.

From the foregoing discussion one should not conclude that the findings of the present study are either relegated to or are best expressed by a factor-analytic approach. Such framework is used here as an example to demonstrate how these findings may be utilized to engender progress and stimulate research in current conceptualizations of mental abilities.

What Is Localization?

Throughout this monograph it can be inferred that both the design of the experiment and the treatment of the data were organized around an effort to localize higher cortical functions. The nature of this effort is discussed here.

The title of this subsection is paraphrased from *Bay* [1964] who stated that the question was not *whether* there is localization but *what is localized and how.* He differentiated between the localizability of simple functions, such as moving a leg, and complex functions (activities of the organism as a whole directed toward a goal) such as jumping over a hurdle. For the latter, he used the German word 'Leistung' which *Conrad* [*Schaltenbrand and Woolsey,* 1964] deemed untranslatable into English. *Bay* translated it as *performance;* I would rather translate it less literally as *process* to emphasize the aspect of the act with which we are most concerned, the ongoing admixture of activity necessary for *performance* to occur. In other words, moving a leg is a simple function while jumping over a hurdle or speaking is a *performance* but more fundamentally a *process.*

Bay enumerated two different approaches toward the problem of localization, one anatomical and the other functional or physiological. He described how the anatomical approach attempts to establish immediate and constant relations between clinical findings and the location of anatomical lesions, and how this approach has proven valid for e.g. motor functions up to and including Broca's aphasia. The discovery of the latter brought about the reification of other cognitive components such as agnosia, apraxia and acalculia which were created quite hypothetically and in strict analogy to aphasia. There is little agreement and very little evidence as to whether these terms have neurophysiological meaning, and they certainly do not constitute neuro-anatomical entities.

As a consequence of this frustration, the search for new cognitive structures has more recently resorted to adopting linguistic terms without getting any closer to the goal. The search was stymied by the handicap of having only one method through which to infer functions, i.e. the study of deficits consequent to lesions. The advantage of the present methodology is that changes in the functional role of brain areas can be inferred from changes in electrocortical activity.

The difference between the two methods is not just in the higher degree of precision obtainable in the latter. There is a fundamental difference between the two and the type of data that they yield. In the deficit studies one is restricted to administering a number of tests to determine the type of deficit present with a lesion in a given brain area. With the present methodology one can study the electrical changes occurring in that same brain area in a healthy brain under a variety of conditions but more importantly one can study the concomitant changes in activity in any number of other brain areas.

As a result EEG spectral analysis as used in the present investigation makes possible the determination of how the performance of a given function involves different regions of the brain. It also makes possible the determination of how two seemingly independent functions are electrophysiologically related. This latter possibility is fundamental in the search for determining functions *à la brain,* i.e. conceptualizing the functions according to neurophysiologically meaningful categories.

Rather than being restricted to, for instance, the evidence of word-finding deficits ensuing from a brain with a given lesion, with the present methodology words can be experimentally and repeatedly administered, searched, heard, read in any number of ways or combinations, and changes can be observed when they occur in any number of scalp positions, all from a healthy functioning brain. In addition, this methodology permits the investigation of whether word-finding should be considered to be an electrophysiologically independent category.

It is now possible to develop a better understanding of how these exquisitely complex functions are performed in this marvelously complex organ, the human brain. Are the mind and brain one? With progress in neuropsychology unparalleled by progress in philosophy are we demonstrating that mind is mostly brain, or are we finding where brain meets the mind? The answers to these questions will have to wait for tomorrow.

References

Adey, W.R.: Spectral analysis of EEG data from animals and man during alerting, orienting and discriminative responses; in Evans, Mulholland, Attention in neurophysiology, pp. 194–229 (Butterworth, London 1969).

Bay, E.: The history of aphasia and the principles of cerebral localization; in Schaltenbrand, Woolsey, Cerebral localization and organization, pp. 43–52 (University of Wisconsin Press, Madison 1964).

Eccles, J.C.; Robinson, D.N.: The wonder of being human (Free Press, New York 1984).

Gasser, T.; Lucadou-Müller, I. von; Verleger, R.; Bächer, P.: Correlating EEG and IQ: a new look at an old problem using computerized EEG parameters. Electroenceph. clin. Neurophysiol. *55:* 493–504 (1983).

Giannitrapani, D.: EEG average frequency and intelligence. Electroenceph. clin. Neurophysiol. *27:* 480–486 (1969).

Giannitrapani, D.: WAIS IQ as related to EEG frequency scores. Electroenceph. clin. Neurophysiol. *28:* 102 (1970).

Giannitrapani, D.: Intelligence and EEG spectra. Electroenceph. clin. Neurophysiol. *34:* 733–734 (1973).

John, E.R.; Ahn, H.; Prichep, L.; Trepetin, M.; Brown, D.; Kaye, H.: Developmental equations for the electroencephalogram. Science *210:* 1255–1258 (1980).

Katada, A.; Ozaki, H.; Suzuki, H.; Suhara, K.: Developmental characteristics of normal and mentally retarded children's EEG. Electroenceph. clin. Neurophysiol. *52:* 192–201 (1981).

Knott, J.R.; Friedman, H.; Bardsley, R.: Some electroencephalographic correlates of intelligence in eight-year and twelve-year-old children. J. exp. Psychol. *30:* 380–391 (1942).

Liberson, W.T.: Ondes électriques du cerveau et intelligence; PhD thesis, Montreal (mimeographed, 1950).

Luria, A.R.: Higher cortical functions in man (Basic Books, New York 1966).

Osaka, M.; Osaka, N.: Human intelligence and power spectral analysis of visual evoked potentials. Percept. Mot. Skills *50:* 192–194 (1980).

Penfield, W.; Roberts, L.: Speech and brain mechanisms (Princeton University Press, Princeton 1959).

Schaltenbrand, G.; Woolsey, C.N.: Cerebral localization and organization, p. 53 (University of Wisconsin Press, Madison 1964).

Wechsler, D.: WISC Manual, Wechsler Intelligence Scale for Children (Psychological Corp., New York 1949).

Weinberg, H.: Correlation of frequency spectra of averaged visual evoked potentials with verbal intelligence. Nature, Lond. *224:* 813–815 (1969).

Glossary

Acalculia. A disorder which affects the facility for manipulating numbers and performing computations.

A/D conversion, cf. Digitizing.

Agnosia. A disturbance characterized by the failure to recognize familiar objects by at least one of the senses.

Agraphia. A disturbance in writing consisting either of the inability to form letters or of defects in language.

Algorithm. A procedure for solving a mathematical problem in a finite number of steps. It may indicate that a solution is not possible.

Alpha activity. A portion of the EEG spectrum in the frequency range from 8 to 12 Hz. It is often incorrectly used in place of dominant alpha activity.

Alpha desynchronization. A feature of the EEG corresponding to an apparent decrease of dominant alpha activity due to the lack of synchronization of individual alpha waves. It occurs often during stimulation. Presumably, synchronized alpha activity is produced by millions of cells and results in the amplitude corresponding to dominant alpha activity.

Alpha frequency, cf. Dominant alpha frequency.

Alpha index (percent time alpha). A measure of the percentage of time in which dominant alpha activity is present during a given EEG period. The difficulty in this measurement is that the criterion of the presence of dominant alpha is determined subjectively.

Analog recording. A system using magnetic tape for recording analog waveforms. There are basically two recording methods for analog signals: amplitude modulation (AM) and frequency modulation (FM), the latter being preferred for a more faithful reproduction of the signals; cf. Frequency modulation.

Analog-to-digital conversion, cf. Digitizing.

Analog wave. A waveform having a continuously changing voltage. Because of this, numerical computations cannot be performed directly and the waveform cannot be entered in a digital computer. Analysis can be performed directly in an analog computer.

Aphasia. A condition consisting of a loss of language functions. More generally, it refers to those motor and sensory language disturbances caused by brain lesions.

Apnea. Breathlessness resulting from many causes, e.g., forced respiration or excess oxygen in the blood.

Apraxia. A disturbance characterized by the inability to perform complex movements upon request.

Autospectrum. Output of Fourier analysis which plots intensity of activity (in the form of power scores) as a function of frequency. Since it consists of an estimate of the frequency content of the original signal, the study of the differences in such content is thus possible.

BCD, cf. Binary coded decimal.

Beat frequency. The frequency at which the envelope of a sinusoidal wave increases or decreases in amplitude as a result of being composed of 2 waves at slightly different frequencies. The beat frequency is equal to the difference between the frequencies of the 2 waves.

Beta activity. EEG activity ranging in frequency from 17 Hz upward. It is often subdivided into low beta (17–23 Hz) and high beta (23 Hz plus).

Binary coded decimal (BCD). A binary format for recording decimal information, requiring 4 bits for representing digits from 0 to 9. It is not the most parsimonious translation of digits from the decimal to the binary system, but when space is not an issue, it presents a certain ease in translation.

Binary information. Information which is recorded in any of the several binary codes; cf. Two's complement or Binary coded decimal.

Brain dominance. The dominance of one of the two brain hemispheres in presiding over the execution of a specific cortical function. It is often incorrectly used to imply the concept of the dominance of a whole hemisphere in presiding over all higher cortical functions. In a right-handed population this would be the left hemisphere.

Broca's area. The first of the brain areas identified as presiding over language functions. Later found to relate to the motor aspects of speech, it is located in the lateral aspect of the frontal lobe anterior to the precentral gyrus, usually in the left hemisphere. It is approximately located between the F_7 and T_3 electrode.

CFF, cf. Critical flicker frequency.

Character. A term of digital technology referring to a set of parallel bits (e.g. simultaneously written on or read from a tape).

Chirality. The study of asymmetries in the development of organisms such as the left-handed or right-handed spirals of snail shells.

Complex waveform. A tracing, such as the EEG, composed of sinusoidal waves of more than one frequency. The purpose of spectral analysis is to identify and measure these frequency components.

Constructional apraxia. A disturbance in the imaging processes reflected in a deficit in constructional activity. It results in the production of an incorrect form from the spatial point of view even though difficulty in the execution of other complex or skilled movements typical of apraxia may not be present.

Contralaterality. Lateralization of functions in the hemisphere opposite to the side of the preferred hand.

Correlation coefficient. A measure of the degree of relationship between two variables. It ranges from 1.0, which indicates that the 2 variables are directly and linearly proportional, to -1.0 which occurs when the 2 variables are inversely and linearly proportional. 0 indicates a random relationship between 2 variables; cf. Pearson r and Spearman rho.

Cortex. The most recently developed portion of the brain which presides over more complex functions. It is the outermost layer, closest to the scalp. All EEG data being derived from scalp electrodes are therefore a reflection of cortical activity subject to modification due to lower brain structures. Because of folding, not all cortical regions can be effectively recorded from scalp electrodes.

Critical flicker frequency (CFF). The frequency at which an intermittent visual stimulus is perceived as barely flickering. If the frequency of the intermittent stimulus is faster, the stimulus does not appear to be flickering.

Cross spectrum. Output of Fourier analysis which permits exploration of the average common-frequency relationships between 2 time series. As such it measures the similarity in the frequency composition of 2 signals originating in 2 points in the scalp.

Cytoarchitecture. The manner in which cells are structurally arranged.

D/A, cf. Digital-to-analog conversion.

D/A conversion, cf. Digital-to-analog conversion.

Decussation. The manner in which neural fibers cross in the brain so that functions on the right side of the body are represented in the left cerebral hemisphere and vice versa. The most important is the corticospinal decussation of the pyramidal tracts. Even though contralateral motor functions had been observed earlier, the first anatomical description and representation of the corticospinal decussation is attributed to Mistichelli in 1709. Decussations are generally partial so that only a percentage of the functions crosses while the remainder remains uncrossed. This percentage varies in the same individual in the left and right sides so that not the same percentage of fibers crosses from left to right as that which crosses from right to left.

Delta activity. EEG activity ranging in frequency up to and including 3 Hz.

Differentiation. A characteristic of embryonic cells to multiply and at the same time to diversify in structure and function. Also the capacity of an organism, during development, to change its response to stimuli from global to specific.

Digital recording. A system using magnetic tape or disc for recording digital signals. Data from these media if recorded in a compatible format, can be entered into a digital computer without additional processing. Performing A/D (analog-to-digital) conversion of electrophysiological signals and recording the conversions at the time of data acquisition permits the storage of electrophysiological data and their direct analysis in a digital computer.

Digital-to-analog conversion (D/A conversion). A process by which a digitized signal is reconstituted in its original analog format. If the original digitization was performed with adequate resolution (i.e. with sufficient numbers of samples per unit time) the reconstituted analog waveform is undistinguishable from the original analog waveform from which it was derived.

Digitizing (analog-to-digital conversion; A/D conversion). A process by which the voltage of an analog signal is measured at regular intervals. The process can be very fast (a million times per second) so that no information is lost. The purpose of digitizing is to permit numerical computations of an analog waveform which has been transformed by this process from an analog variable into a discrete variable.

Dominant activity, cf. Dominant alpha activity.

Dominant alpha activity. The portion of alpha activity which has much greater amplitude and regularity than the other frequencies in that range. It is usually found to be of higher amplitude in occipital or parietal areas during awake resting with eyes closed. Not all individuals show dominant alpha activity, and the correlates of its presence are not known. In its purest form it appears as an almost perfect sinusoid and as such represents along with sleep spindles one of the more esthetically pleasing activities of the EEG spectrum.

Dominant alpha frequency (alpha frequency). The frequency constituting the waveform of dominant alpha activity in a given subject.

EEG, cf. Electroencephalogram.

EEG driving. A phenomenon whereby certain EEG frequencies (primarily alpha activity) can increase in amplitude when the organism is exposed to a stimulus (primarily visual) having a frequency equal or near to the EEG frequency which is being driven.

Electroencephalogram (EEG). Literally, the electric writing of the head. The first use of the technique in its present form is attributed to *Berger* [1929, cf. *Gloor,* 1969]. While the nature of electrical activity in single neurons is fairly well understood, it is not clear whether the EEG is the resultant of synchronous firing of millions of neurons or of changes in electrical fields only indirectly related to the firings of these neurons.

Electronic averaging. The algebraic summation of 2 or more waveforms so that 2 positive voltages are added and a positive and a negative voltage are subtracted from each other. When the summation is performed on signals having a common stimulus trigger, the electronic averaging permits the emergence of common features of the signals which follow the trigger stimulus; cf. Evoked potentials.

Equal intervals. In the computation of correlation the Pearson r formula assumes equality between the intervals of the numerical progression used. This assumption cannot be made for psychological variables when numerical values are given to responses to questions. Since the absolute difficulty of the items cannot be measured, the scores represent a numerical progression without any assumption of linearity. In this case the use of a rank-order correlation formula is more appropriate; cf. Spearman rho.

Evoked potentials. That portion of EEG activity, usually buried in noise, which becomes apparent through electronic averaging and which results from a specific kind of stimulation.

Factor. The end-product of factor analysis. It consists of a mathematically derived variable whose content is more homogeneous and unitary than empirically derived variables. Factors are always a function of the variables introduced in the analysis and are defined by their loadings; cf. Factor loadings. The name given to a factor is a result of speculation as it is based on the evaluation of the magnitude of the loadings that each experimental variable contributes to the factor.

Factor analysis. A multivariate analysis technique developed by Spearman for analyzing the structure of covariance or correlation matrices. The aim of factor analysis is the explanation of relationships among numerous correlated variables in terms of a relatively few underlying variables or factors; cf. Factor and Factor loadings.

Factor loadings. Coefficients of relationship between the original variables and the derived factors. They are the components of the factor matrix resulting from a factor analysis.

Factor rotation. A step in the computation of factor analysis which involves the mathematical rotation of principal component factors. It is the process of redefining the factor axes so that they represent the original variables in a statistically more significant way.

Factor scores. Scores obtained for a given individual representing the value attributed to him for that factor. They are obtained by applying the loadings of that factor on a certain variable to the individual subject's score on that variable. The composite of all the loading computations made for all pertinent variables for that factor constitutes the score for that individual for that factor. They can then be used in the same manner as scores obtained from individual variables.

Fast Fourier transform [reported in its present form by *Cooley and Tukey,* 1965]. An algorithm for the computation of Fourier coefficients which facilitates spectral analysis because of great computational efficiency; cf. Fourier analysis.

FM, cf. Frequency modulation.

Fourier analysis (used here synonymously with spectral analysis and frequency analysis). A mathematical procedure which performs the transformation of data points from the time domain into the frequency domain by fitting the time domain points with a sum of harmonically related sine and cosine waves.

Frequency analysis, cf. Fourier analysis.

Frequency modulation (FM). A preferred method of recording electrophysiological signals in their analog format. Despite common belief, FM recording is still subject to relatively large errors, especially when analyzing the data involves repetitive playback. For this reason FM recording was not used in this study.

Glioma. A rapidly growing tumor of cerebral tissue.

Harmonics. Sinusoidal waveforms at frequencies which are integral multiples of a basic frequency called the fundamental or first harmonic. In sound, the harmonics are primarily responsible for the qualitative differences in the same note rendered by different instruments.

Hippocampus. A portion of the archicortex buried in the temporal lobe in man.

Homologous areas. Brain areas which correspond symmetrically in the left and right cerebral hemispheres. In the precentral gyrus they represent motor functions in grossly symmetrical parts of the body.

Hyperspace, cf. Orthogonal.

Hz. Abbreviation for Hertz (German physicist) representing a unit of measure for the frequency of sinusoidal waveforms. It is synonymous with cycle per second (cps or c/s).

Intelligence quotient (IQ). A standardized scoring method developed by Wechsler for measuring intelligence. For each age group the score is standarized to a mean = 100 and a $\sigma = 15$. In a normal distribution a score of 90 would fall at a point equal to -1 probable error of the mean (-1 PE = lower quartile), so that the scores between 90 and 110 include 50% of the population; cf. Mental age and Z score.

Kappa activity. An EEG rhythm in the theta and alpha frequency bands which increases in amplitude with thinking.

Lateralization. An asymmetrical distribution of functions in the two cortical hemispheres. Use of the term avoids the connotation of whole hemisphere dominance which is often included with the use of the term 'brain dominance'.

Left preferent. An individudal for whom the left side of the body is more dominant than the right, i.e. who prefers the left side of the body over the right. In general, synonymous with left-handed but used instead of the latter to avoid two often implied assumptions: (1) that the hand is representative of the dominance of the entire side of the body and (2) that left and right dominance consists of a dichotomous variable.

Matrix. As used in this study, an array of values ordered in rows (brain areas) and columns (frequency bands).

Mental abilities (mental faculties). The capacity for performing functions which are subsumed under the general category of intelligence. Their measurement is attempted by including a variety of subtests in an intelligence test. They can be regarded as traits, but the term is often used synonymously with intelligence.

Mental age. An early attempt at defining different levels of intelligence based on the calibration of abilities which children at different ages are expected on the average to attain. It was used in the early definition of IQ which was computed as mental age/chronological age. This formula incorrectly assumes a linear relationship between mental age and chronological age.

Mental faculties, cf. Mental abilities.

Mesencephalon (midbrain). The short portion of the brain between the pons and the cerebral hemispheres.

μV, cf. Microvolt.

Microvolt (μV). A measure of amplitude of an EEG signal corresponding to 1,000,000th of a volt (10^{-6} V). Average EEG signals reach an amplitude of from 50 to 100 μV, and dominant alpha activity may reach an amplitude of 200 μV. Paroxysmal activity may reach 500 μV and up.

Midbrain, cf. Mesencephalon.

Neocortex. The more common and phylogenetically more recent structure found on the outer surfaces of the cerebral hemispheres. It consists of six layers of cells which have their embryologic origin in the gray matter surrounding the ventricles.

Nyquist frequency. The minimum sampling rate required for the purpose of digitizing a signal to perform Fourier analysis. It is equal to twice the highest frequency present in the data whether or not that high frequency is of analytic interest. This requirement guarantees that each wave is sampled at least twice. While this requirement is satisfactory for a complex waveform having components which are stationary, it is not necessarily adequate for a signal having components which are continuously changing. As a consequence, poor resolution of that signal will result.

Off line. A method which specifies that the execution of a process, analysis or computer program is performed subsequent to the data acquisition, generally through the use of a playback of the recorded data. This often occurs when the process is too time-consuming to keep pace with the data acquisition process.

On line. A method which specifies that the execution of a process, analysis or computer program is performed simultaneously with the data acquisition.

One-tailed test. A test of statistical significance used when the investigator has an explicit hypothesis concerning the direction of the difference between the compared scores.

Ontogenesis. The developmental changes of the individual. These changes can grossly be considered to recapitulate phylogenesis.

Orthogonal. Here referring to statistically independent factor vectors. More than 3 orthogonal factors cannot be represented visually, in which case postulating spaces of greater than 3 dimensions (hyperspace) can assist in conceptualizing the factors.

Parameter. A set of physical properties whose values determine the characteristics of a variable.

Pearson r. A measure of association indicating the strength of the linear relationship between two variables. This common correlation coefficient is expressed as

$$r = \Sigma xy / \sqrt{\Sigma x^2 \Sigma y^2}; \text{ cf. Correlation coefficient.}$$

Pearson r². A measure of association concerned with the strength of the relationship between two variables. It is a measure of the proportion of variance in one variable explained by the other.

Percent time alpha, cf. Alpha index.

Period. The time needed for a sinusoidal wave to complete one full cycle. It corresponds to the reciprocal of the wave's frequency.

Periodicity. The characteristic of a signal of repeating cyclically the same sequence of values.

Phonemic. Pertaining to a group of closely similar speech sounds regarded in a given language as being the same sound.

Phylogenesis. A developmental process whereby more primitive, lower-order species (phyla) evolve into more advanced organisms.

Plasticity. An attribute of living tissue stronger in the embryo and young organsims. It consists of the ability of cells to change function due to causes internal (e.g. development) or external (e.g. injury or trauma) to the organism.

Power scores. Scores resulting from a Fourier analysis. They are proportional to the square of the amplitude (voltage) of a signal in given frequency bands.

Power spectral density. The frequency composition of a complex waveform such as the EEG. Since the waveform analyzed is not of infinite length, the spectral values obtained are estimates of the power (amplitude squared) which occurs in the various frequency bands.

Pyramidal tracts. The primary motor fibers which control voluntary movements of skeletal muscles. They project on the cortex in the primary motor area of the precentral gyrus (Brodman area 4). The name derives from the presence of giant pyramidal (Betz) cells. The precentral gyrus is probably partially intersected by the central electrode placements in the study.

Refractory period. The length of time during which a neuron, after firing a spike, cannot fire another spike regardless of the magnitude of stimulation. The greatest portion of the effect lasts no more than 100 ms.

Reliability. A statistic designed to measure the degree of variation or error of a score over time. Since the Pearson r^2 between 2 EEG signals is an estimate of the variance accounted for by the correlation between them, it can be used as an estimate of the reliability or predictability of the signal.

Rho, cf. Spearman rho.

Right preferent. An individual for whom the right side of the body is more dominant than the left, i.e., who prefers the right side of the body to the left. In general, synonymous with right-handed but used instead of the latter to avoid two often implied assumptions: (1) that the hand is representative of the dominance of the entire side of the body and (2) that right and left dominance consists of a dichotomous variable.

Sampling rate. The rate at which the voltage of a wave is measured (i.e., the amplitude of a signal is digitized).

Signal-to-noise ratio. The ratio (in decibels on a logarithmic scale) between the signal being recorded (at its maximum amplitude) and the noise level of the system. It is used as a measure of the dynamic range (frequency range) of a recording system. In EEG the fluctuating nature of the signals, having a significant portion of the recording at minimum amplitude, should be taken into account when estimating the signal-to-noise ratio.

Source trait. An underlying influence or factor assumed to be the determinant of overt behavior. Since it is not necessarily directly observable in behavior it may be detectable via indirect methods such as factor analysis.

Spearman rho. A measure of correlation which makes no assumption about the distribution of the two variables. It is a rank order correlation because it is computed from each subject's rank on the two variables rather than from the computation of actual scores as is the case in the computation of the Pearson r.

$$\text{rho} = 1 - \frac{6\Sigma d^2}{N(N^2 - 1)} \quad \text{where } d = \Sigma \text{ Ranks } (x_i) - \Sigma \text{ Ranks } (y_i).$$

Spectral analysis, cf. Fourier analysis.

Standard score, cf. Z score.

Stationarity. An attribute of a signal which even though regarded as a random process has a frequency composition homogeneous in subsequent periods of time. The length of the time period used for an analysis can thus determine whether the signal is effectively stationary.

Steady-state EEG. The complex waveform produced by the brain during a homogeneous behavioral state, as distinguished from evoked potentials.

Surface trait. A trait or quality as it appears in overt behavior. It can be inferred from a cluster of correlations which indicate that certain variables are related to each other in a manifest way.

Theta activity. EEG activity ranging in frequency from 4 to 7 Hz.

Two's complement. One of the most parsimonious formats for recording numerical information in binary form. While a 4-bit character can represent digits from 0 to 9 in BCD format, it can represent numbers from 0 to 15 in 2's complement format.

Two-tailed test. A test of statistical significance used when the investigator does not have an explicit hypothesis concerning the expected direction of the difference between the compared scores. It is a more conservative test of significance than the one-tailed test.

Wernicke's area. A brain area alleged to be associated with the ideational aspect of speech. It is often referred to as the posterior speech area. Damage in that area may produce a failure to understand language and also a propensity for producing speech devoid of content. It is located in a region posterior to the T_3 electrode and broadly across the distance between P_3 and T_5.

Z score (standard score). A transformation of raw scores related to the mean and standard deviation of a distribution. $z = (X - \overline{X})/\sigma$. Such transformation permits direct comparison of scores from distributions having different means and standard deviations. IQ scores are z scores with the mean = 100 and the σ = 15.

Author Index

Subject Index

THIS VOLUME MAY CIRCULATE FOR 2 WEEKS
Renewals May Be Made In Person Or By Phone:

66050   x 5300; from outside 472-5300
746-6050

DATE DUE	DATE RETURNED
DEC 9 1985 W	
Dec. 21	1985 W
JUN 4 1986 FM	JUN. 3 1986
OCT 2 0 1986 W	OCT. 2 0 1986
MAY 29 1991 B	

99427